AIDS, FEAR, AND SOCIETY

AIDS, FEAR, AND SOCIETY

Challenging the Dreaded Disease

Kenneth J. Doka
Graduate School
College of New Rochelle
New Rochelle, New York

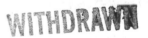

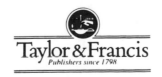
Taylor & Francis
Publishers since 1798

362.19697
1658a
1997

USA	Publishing Office:	Taylor & Francis 1101 Vermont Avenue, NW, Suite 200 Washington, DC 20005-3521 Tel: (202) 289-2174 Fax: (202) 289-3665
	Distribution Center:	Taylor & Francis 1900 Frost Road, Suite 101 Bristol, PA 19007-1598 Tel: (215) 785-5800 Fax: (215) 785-5515
UK		Taylor & Francis Ltd. 1 Gunpowder Square London EC4A 3DE Tel: 171 583 0490 Fax: 171 583 0581

AIDS, FEAR, AND SOCIETY: Challenging the Dreaded Disease

1 2 3 4 5 6 7 8 9 0   B R B R   9 8 7

This book was set in Times Roman. The editor was Catherine Simon. Cover design by Michelle Fleitz. Bottom photo (group of men) © David Ryan, 1990, PNI.

A CIP catalog record for this book is available from the British Library.
∞ The paper in this publication meets the requirements of the ANSI Standard Z39.48-1984 (Permanence of Paper)

Library of Congress Cataloging-in-Publication Data

Doka, Kenneth J.
  AIDS, fear, and society: challenging the dreaded disease/
Kenneth J. Doka.
      p.   cm.—(Series in death education, aging, and health care,
ISSN 0275-3510)
  Includes bibliographical references.
  1. AIDS (Disease)—Social aspects. 2. AIDS (Disease)—History.
3. Epidemiology. I. Title. II. Series.
RA644.A25D65   1997
362.1'969792—dc20   96-44899
                                                            CIP

ISBN 1-56032-248-9 (cloth)
ISBN 1-56032-681-6 (paper)
ISSN 0275-3510

To
Michael Whitehead
and all who have died from
dreaded diseases
and to
Linda and Keith Whitehead
and all who were touched
by their deaths and lives

CONTENTS

Part I
NATURE, HISTORY, AND RESPONSES
TO DREADED DISEASES

FOREWORD

In "The Stuff of Life," an installation-style linocut by Eric Avery, the viewer is assaulted by enormously magnified cells from a human blood smear—one that might be used to test for HIV. We find ourselves at once immersed in both the cosmic and the microscopic, our universe of healthy blood cells being threatened by ominous virus spheres. The larger-than-life work becomes a reminder of the insidious threat of AIDS and the need to look beyond the microscope to make sense of it.

"The Stuff of Life" is important for two reasons: It is activist art and, paradoxically, healing art as well. As an artist, practicing physician, and AIDS psychiatrist, Eric Avery employs art as a vehicle for containing and releasing the tension he experiences in his daily encounters with patients and the medical system.

The healing power of art has long been recognized by such diverse cultures as the Navajo, Tibetan Buddhists, and Christian mystics. Sand paintings, "chants," mantras, and visualizations in some way or other require a blending or absorption of the healing properties from both spiritual and environmental sources. As "medicine," these media rely on the relationships among mind, body, spirit, and even community.

Building on these traditions, Avery takes art and the concept of healing spaces one step further. He turns the table. Addressing the ethical ramifications of AIDS, he challenges physicians and health care bureaucrats to venture beyond the safety of familiar hospital settings to bring themselves and their armamentarium of syringes, tests, and counseling skills into the most unlikely of public places—galleries and museums. The mantra of medical ethics—benevolence, nonmalfeasance, autonomy, and justice—is abruptly catapulted from the realm of theory to that of praxis.

The gauntlet Eric Avery threw down in the medical/arts arena has been taken up in the sociohistoric realm by Ken Doka. Clergy person, sociologist, teacher, and counselor, Doka has chosen to tackle the topic of dread diseases—in particular, AIDS—in the larger contexts of history, sociology, and religion. Viewing AIDS alongside such other historical "plagues" as syphilis, leprosy, tuberculosis, and cancer, Doka engages us with the stories of human beings living with these chronic, disfiguring, debilitating illnesses. Rather than focusing on statistics and the biological ravages produced by the various maladies, Doka directs our attention instead to concerns about quality of life. In so doing, he underscores the human dimensions of his thesis as he debates the antithetical issues of public health and private morality. As in his two earlier books, *Living with Life-Threatening Illness: A Guide for Patients, Their Families, and Caregivers* (1993) and *Disenfranchised Grief: Recognizing Hidden Sorrow* (1989), this current work attests to his vast experience in both scholarly and clinical settings.

In a wonderfully readable style, each chapter presents concise overviews of various illnesses, delineates the moral dimensions of epidemics, and spells out the ways in which attitudes toward and assumptions about dreaded diseases have, in turn, changed the nature of the societies they afflicted. The reader becomes sensitized to the inherent tension between the rights of the individuals affected and those of society as a whole.

Doka supports his contentions with both traditional metaphors and fresh insights. Take, for example, the sharing of needles by intravenous drug users. Reminding us of the significance of blood and its use in rituals of purification, community, and covenants, Doka helps us appreciate the more subtle nuances of needle-sharing beyond the economic and addictive elements.

Doka's book not only educates us, but, like Avery's work, challenges us to "walk the talk," so to speak. In addition, Doka furnishes us with the tools, the critical facts and understanding, to enable our patients and friends to become their own advocates as well as the ammunition to advocate for them in deed and policy. With such tentative progress being made in the fight against AIDS and the increasing number of people afflicted by it, we owe the author a debt of gratitude for broadening our perspectives and transforming paralysis and helplessness in the face of this dreaded disease to promise, hope, and action.

Sandra L. Bertman, Ph.D.
Professor of Humanities in Medicine
University of Massachusetts Medical Center

PREFACE

It is rumored that the disease is spread by design by external enemies in order to weaken the nation.

Other rumors suggest that internal opponents have introduced the disease or aided its spread to decimate a stigmatized and marginalized group.

Still other rumors hold that those with the disease are actively seeking to spread it to healthy populations so that they may share in the misery.

To some the disease has a clear theological message, a warning to populations to turn from their sins. Others see it as a judgment on society for failing to alleviate poverty or tolerating vice.

The disease itself stigmatizes victims: Many are driven from their homes, abhorred by their families, or refused treatment by hospitals.

Even in death, the disease carries a sense of dread. Families are reluctant to admit the cause of death.

It may seem surprising as one reads the above statements that the diseases described are not AIDS. AIDS, or acquired immune deficiency syndrome, is just one of a series of dreaded diseases that have aroused both great fear and irrational actions. Throughout history, a variety of diseases (bubonic plague, tuberculosis, syphilis, and cholera, to name a few) have evoked the above responses and, much like AIDS today, created such a sense of dread that rational moves to halt the disease were compromised. In all of these cases the fear overwhelmed.

Many readers can remember the fear that cancer caused less than a generation ago. One incident stays in my mind. When I was a young boy, we had tenants in our two-family house with whom I was especially close. Every day I would visit with "Aunt" Francis and "Uncle" Walter. When I was small, Aunt

Francis used to read stories to me from a big picture book that she had bought to read for her children, now grown. Aunt Francis developed cancer. When she left the house for what she knew would be her last hospitalization, she gave me that book. When I looked for it later, I learned that one of my aunts had thrown it out. When I confronted this aunt, she resolvedly defended her action. After all, she reminded my parents, you just never know.

Susan Sontag's two seminal works, *Illness as Metaphor* (1978) and *AIDS and Its Metaphors* (1988), remind us that people's metaphors about disease reflect and frame the ways they perceive disease. And the way people perceive disease influences the ways they respond to persons with that disease.

One central point of this book is that AIDS strikes a deep primal fear. AIDS has become the archetype of all the dreaded diseases that have troubled humankind throughout its history. This fear, this sense of dread, has done to the present society what it has done in the past. The deep sense of fear that AIDS evokes has stigmatized those who suffer from the disease as well as their families and caregivers. It has marginalized those populations perceived to be most at risk. It has politicized AIDS so badly that rational discussions of what might be effective public health and preventive measures have become virtually impossible. Until AIDS is looked at in the same way as other life-threatening illnesses, rather than steeped in fear, society will be inhibited from developing policies and practices that will stem the disease and provide for humane treatment of persons suffering from, or at least at risk for, AIDS.

The book emphasizes another critical point: Diseases are more than biological phenomena or individual catastrophes. They are profoundly social events. In many cases, the disease emerges and spreads because changing social conditions trouble the fragile balances that exist between humans and their diseases. In other situations, a disease is perceived or recognized in a distinct way, reflecting new social conditions and forces. In all cases, the ways in which a disease is spread and treated are strongly influenced by larger sociological considerations. And the emergence of new, or newly perceived, diseases is likely to change social institutions and perhaps society itself.

In order to understand the fears generated by AIDS and the effects that it has, it is necessary to root AIDS in the history of diseases that also struck such a chord of fear and so influenced their societies. This allows one to see how, in the past, fear inhibited humane and effective control and treatment of diseases. Part I reviews the nature and history of those earlier dreaded diseases and society's responses to them.

The dreaded diseases were of two types. One was the great epidemics that periodically devastated societies. The second type was stigmatized diseases such as syphilis, leprosy, or cancer. These diseases did not cause the collective devastation of the epidemic plagues, but they did condemn individuals to death characterized by agony, pain, and isolation. Although these disease types were different, and had different effects, both evoked a sense of dread that inhibited sufferers from seeking and receiving help. In both types of dreaded diseases, the very actions intended to halt or slow the spread of disease frequently exacerbated the spread.

Part II considers AIDS as the archetype of the dreaded disease. AIDS (or human immunodeficiency virus [HIV] infection) shares characteristics of both types of dreaded disease described above. One can see how AIDS has created a sense of panic and fear that haunts current policy and practice. AIDS, too, is a social disease, emerging from changes in the social order and likely to have significant effects on that order.

Hannelore Wass (1986), early in the epidemic, wrote of AIDS, "the disease has a *potential* for becoming an epidemic; the fear of AIDS already *is* a major epidemic" (original emphasis; p. xii). AIDS has the potential for becoming a major scourge of humankind, perhaps as devastating as the plague, perhaps, as some have suggested, a species killer. But AIDS presents another danger. Like the dreaded diseases of the past, it can unleash fears that can tear the very fabric of society. There is a parable that expresses this well: It seems a traveler came across the plague as it was on its way to Baghdad. Questioned, the plague announced it would slay five thousand in the city. Meeting the plague again on the return, the traveler challenged it: "You said you would slay but five thousand, yet fifty thousand died." The plague answered, "I did as I said, only five thousand did I kill. The rest were killed by fear." The only hope of halting the AIDS epidemic is to contain the epidemic of fear and control the irrationality it begets.

ACKNOWLEDGMENTS

One of the greatest pleasures in completing a work is to acknowledge those who have helped make the idea a reality. As with any creation, so many have left their marks, in one way or another, on this book.

My colleagues in the Association for Death Education and Counseling (ADEC) and the International Work Group on Death, Dying, and Bereavement (IWG) have been continued sources of intellectual stimulation and personal support. So many have helped in so many ways that it seems unfair to single out just a few. Some, however, do call for special acknowledgment: Robert Fulton, Van Pine, and Robert Kastenbaum have always been my mentors. The first two have encouraged my sociological perspective whereas the latter has always urged me in more clinical directions. Hannelore Wass also deserves special mention. This book, in many respects, reflects her vision. Sandra Bertman, Charles Corr, and John Morgan have also left their subtle marks on these pages. In addition, throughout the years Therese A. Rando, Catherine Sanders, Dana Cable, Terry Martin, Jane Nichols, Lu Redmond, Neil Heflin-Wells, Judith Stillion, Tom Attig, Dennis Klass, John Stephenson, Ben Wolfe, Robert Neimeyer, Lynn DeSpelder, Al Strickland, Lois Dick, Donna O'Toole, Earl Grollman, and Betty Murray have been there to provide encouragement and support, as have many of my colleagues at ADEC and IWG. To mention them all would require an entire second volume to this work. Jack Gordon, Norman Sherman, and Dave Abrams of the Hospice Foundation of America have also provided numerous opportunities in the past years for me to grow and develop.

I have received rich support from my institution. The College of New Rochelle has provided one of those enviable "publish and prosper" environments. I want to thank them for the opportunities I have had—to teach, to learn, to grow. I want to thank our administration—President Dorothy Ann Kelly, Vice President Stephen Sweeny, Dean Laura Ellis, and Division Chairs Marguerite Coke and Jerri Frantzve—for creating and nurturing that environment. My colleagues too are part of that positive environment. Those in my division—Robert Arko, Claire Lavin, James Magee, and Dennis Ryan—deserve special mention.

The College of New Rochelle has been generous in technical support as well. Our division secretary, Rosemary Strobel, always manages to do the impossible. Robin Alexander, Jen Ryan, Maura Curry, Vera Mezzaucella, Chris Troeunier, and James Cardali all have helped with various parts of the manuscript. And Carole Polony volunteered to do editing. This was a special gift.

I also must acknowledge the tremendous patience and support of the Taylor & Francis staff. Ron Wilder supported this project from its earliest days. Even in his move to another position, he continued to be helpful. His successor, Elaine Pirrone, followed in that vein. She always had thoughtful suggestions as well as a gentle way of prodding me to completion.

I also need to recognize the assistance of my family. My son, Michael, completed college during the work on this book. It has been interesting discussing ideas and thoughts with him. I have been blessed with many special friends who have offered both respite and stimulation. Kathy, Rick, Kurt, Jill, Jim, and Irene— you all helped me in so many ways. My neighbors, too—Jim and Mary, Paul and Margot, Herb and Terry, Don and Carol, as well as former neighbors Donna, Ted, and Judy—have provided rich support. Watching my godson, Keith, grow and develop also provided special joy. And how could I not acknowledge my parents, my sister Dot, my brother Frank, and their families.

And finally, I want to recognize the many people I have known—some for a long time, others for brief moments—who have died from AIDS. I hope that by making this disease less dreaded, the suffering of all those who may be infected with or affected by this illness may be eased.

PART I
NATURE, HISTORY, AND RESPONSES TO DREADED DISEASES

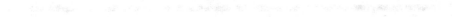

Chapter 1

CRISIS AND CONTAGION

And behold, a pale horse, and its rider's name was death.
Revelation 6:8

THE GREAT EPIDEMICS: AN OVERVIEW

The Black Death or Bubonic Plague

The fourth horse of the apocalypse, the pale one, represents plague. For much of history, disease and epidemic were almost synonymous terms and dreaded for that very reason.

Historically, dreaded diseases have been of two types. The first type is the great epidemics. It is not hard to understand the great sense of dread surrounding epidemics that have swept through the world from time to time. The epidemics have included the great pandemics of bubonic plague (6th and 13th centuries, 1894–1902) and influenza (1918–1919) and the intermittent epidemics of these same diseases or other diseases such as yellow fever, typhus, typhoid, and cholera. The collective devastation of these diseases inspires awesome dread. For example, the mortality rate in Europe during the 1347–1350 epidemic of the plague has been estimated to be between 25 and 75% (Winslow, 1943). The 1894 epidemic of that disease killed more than 13 million eastern Europeans from 1918 to 1922. The influenza epidemic of 1918–1919 led to the loss of more than 700,000 lives. In Philadelphia alone, 12,162 people succumbed to influenza in the weeks between September 29 and November 2.

3

These mortality rates, overwhelming as they are, do not convey the social and corporate devastation that these diseases wrought. These diseases wiped out families and communities. They profoundly altered social institutions. They were epochal events that altered the very course of history. The bubonic plague provides many examples of this. The emphasis on judgmental theology that emerged from the plague's Cult of Death later contributed to the reaction of the Protestant Reformation. The plague also provoked peasant revolts and widespread religious programs that set the stage for ghettoizing Jews (Tuchman, 1978), and social movements of self-flagellants challenged all principles of medieval order.

The bubonic plague would head most lists of these epidemic dreaded diseases. Bubonic plague has two forms. In the more common bubonic form, the infective bacterium (*Pasteurella pestis*, also known as *Yersinia pestis*) affects rats. The fleas carried by the rats can also feed on humans and are apt to do so when the rat population is decimated by disease. Hence, a rat epidemic usually precedes the human one.

The symptoms of plague usually begin with swollen lymph glands in the armpits, neck, and groin. The Greek word for groin, buboes, gave name to the plague. High temperatures, chills, and severe prostration follow the swelling. Death often comes rapidly, within a few days, generally due to septicemia and internal bleeding. It is estimated that in the early epidemics, perhaps between 60 and 90% of those infected died.

The other form of bubonic plague is pneumonic. This form was even more deadly than the bubonic form, with a mortality rate that, in the early years, was well over 90%. The disease progresses as follows: The person's lungs are infected with the bacilli. The disease then can be spread directly from person to person, through spit or air droplets in an infected person's breath. Often this variety has had a large role in major pandemics that have scourged humankind.

Like many early diseases, the roots of the plague are somewhat lost in historical mist. It is suspected that the disease may have emerged somewhere in Central Asia. Some have suggested that the plague of Thucydides may have been bubonic, although most historians believe it was more likely measles, typhus, or fungus ergotism (Marks & Beatty, 1976). In any case, as Marks (1976) concluded, that plague is difficult to identify. Others see bubonic plague as the Old Testament disease that destroyed the Philistines or ended Sennacherib's siege of Jerusalem.

However, these early instances are unclear. It is generally accepted that bubonic plague was the plague of Justinian that swept through Europe and Asia in 541 A.D. Justinian, the Byzantine emperor at that time, was poised to reestablish Rome. He had established peace with Persia, his chief enemy, and his other enemies were divided and weak. He had recaptured Italy from the Ostrogoths and North Africa from the Vandals. The Mediterranean nations seemed to welcome the security and peace his empire could offer. Another era of "pax Romana" or a Byzantine peace seemed at hand. Ironically, it was likely that this very peace facilitated the plague. The peace reopened and extended trade routes through the East and West. Traders and soldiers now had even greater mobility. The changing social conditions allowed the plague the same mobility that would have been inhibited and constrained in a more fragmented world. The dream of a new pax Romana would give way to a new nightmare.

It is estimated that 50% of the population, perhaps as many as 100 million people, died (Marks & Beatty, 1976). In the half century of the disease, whole towns, villages, and even cities disappeared, some never to recover. Agriculture regressed to a subsistence level. Taxes ceased to be paid, diminishing a once full treasury. Large estates were distributed as salary to soldiers, establishing a new social order. A once nascent empire fell into decline, later allowing Egypt and Syria to slip into the Islamic orbit.

Beyond the end of a perhaps renewed empire, the disease influenced the course of history in other ways. It hastened the decline of Greek and Roman medicine, which seemed powerless to stop the epidemic. The ideas of medicine, emerging at the time, that disease was caused by pathogenic agents was discredited. Instead, it was accepted that the disease was divine punishment for heresy's sin and vice. Which heresy was arguable. The emperor, Justinian, spared from the disease, became convinced that Roman theological perspective on the dual nature of Christ, both truly divine and human, was heretical. The Orthodox Roman Church blamed Justinian's perspective that Christ was solely divine as the blasphemy that merited divine punishment. In any case, the plague spurred a populace away from medicine, which seemed so unhelpful, to the church, which would now minister to both body and soul.

Most pandemics, especially the bubonic plague, are self-limiting. Over time, the rat and human populations become too limited to provide a reservoir for the disease. Those who survive may develop total or partial immunity. In northern climates, the hibernation or death of fleas in winter breaks the cycle of transmission.

Thus, after close to 50 years, the plague of Justinian faded as a major health threat. But the plague struck again some eight centuries later. This is not atypical in great epidemics. In their rapid spread, whole populations are exposed to the disease. Many die, but those who are not infected or recover seem to have some immunity. The disease then wanes for lack of a host, perhaps to strike at some future time, when conditions are again favorable for the disease to spread.

Interestingly, the plague seemed to have disappeared from Europe for close to 500 years. Somehow, the transmission chain of rats and fleas and humans had been broken in Europe, though the plague maintained a reservoir in central Asia. McNeill (1976) suggested that the disease might have reemerged in China in 1331, killing as much as half the population (Garrett, 1994), perhaps spreading from Yünnan to Burma through Mongol travelers. From there it was carried to Europe through caravans, affecting both human and rodent conditions.

Social conditions were once again favorable to the spread of the disease. Trade and shipping dramatically increased for a number of reasons. Western naval forces had wrestled the Strait of Gibraltar from Moslem forces that had inhibited Christian ships. New designs in ships allowed safer travel. Unfortunately, rats too were exchanged in addition to goods. And the expanding trade led to increases in the population of the port cities. The growth of cities provided new ecological niches for rats and brought together high densities of people in unhygienic conditions. Bathing was considered unhealthy, fleas and lice a normal part of life. Sewer systems were nonexistent and primitive. Homes made with thatched roofs allowed nesting for rodents and other vermin. These developing urban areas then provided perfect opportunities for diseases to spread, especially one spread by flea-infected rats. Even efforts to contain the disease, such as burning homes of victims, were counterproductive because they simply drove infected rats to seek new shelter.

The plague's initial entry into Europe seems to have been the more direct result of refugees. As reported by one disputed witness, the origins of the 14th century plague seem to have been a primitive form of bacterial warfare. During a siege of Kaffa, a Crimean city now called Theodosia or Feodosiya, the besieging Tartars were struck by a deadly disease. The corpses of these dead soldiers were catapulted into the city, spreading the disease and ending the siege. The survivors of the siege, as well as that of another infected city, fled by ship to other cities, thereby bringing plague in their wake. However dramatic this occurrence, the plague was able to continue to spread through trade routes.

From 1346 to 1361, it is estimated that more than 27 million people died. Most estimates are that 25–40% of the population was killed, although some estimates are even higher (McNeill, 1976; Winslow, 1943).

Again, in the absence of a credible science, the plague, at that point called "The Black Death," was blamed on divine retribution. The disease was perceived as punishment, perhaps for sexual indiscretions or tolerating heresy. A call for a pilgrimage to Rome in 1348 by Pope Clement VI brought more than a million people to Rome, carrying disease as they traveled. Flagellants, religious devotees who whipped themselves for atonement, also marched in processions from town to town, bringing the disease with them. Other forms of obsessiveness, a dancing mania and a widespread cult of the dead, were also common. The disease also caused widespread persecution, most particularly of the Jews but also cripples and lepers. In fact Boswell (1980), in a history of homosexuality, considered the 12th century a tolerant one. Monarchs openly engaged in gay love affairs. Yet there was far less tolerance in the 13th and 14th centuries. There were a number of reasons for this, Boswell believes. The Crusades had heightened religious feelings. The development of nation states and absolute monarchies fed pressures for conformity. But the plague also played a role, buttressing a sense of divine retribution that made all minorities—Jews, lepers, cripples, heretics, and homosexuals—suspect.

The Black Death was an epochal event. Hourani (1991) viewed the plague as a significant factor in Islamic society, depopulating cities and reducing its agricultural base so that it was less prepared for Christian counterattacks that allowed the reconquest of Spain and Ottoman capture of the Islamic world. Others have debated its effects on the West. Some have seen the Black Death as contributing to an emergent individualism (Aires, 1987) and a decline of feudalism (Claster, 1982). It may have unwittingly set the stage for the Reformation, providing Catholicism with a serene judgmental theology that Luther, over a century later, would attack. In any case, it decimated the intellectual classes, particularly those in medicine and the clergy, who were on the caregiving forefront of the epidemic, and turned the philosophical optimism of the 13th century to a deepening sense of doom (A. M. Campbell, 1966).

Most historians believe that the Black Death was a bubonic plague, particularly its more virulent pneumonic form. In this disease, massive internal hemorrhaging caused a black discoloration that may have given the disease its name.[1] However, this perspective has been challenged by Twigg (1984), who argued that the rat–flea–human cycle could not account for the widespread course of the disease and its massive toll. He further suggested that the pneumonic form of the

---

[1]Ziegler (1969) suggested that the term is actually a too-literal translation of the Latin *atra*, which generally means "terrible" or "dreadful," but could be translated as "black."

disease could exist only in certain conditions that were not widespread at the time. Twigg (1984) concluded that the Black Death was not the bubonic plague at all, but a form of anthrax.

Whether this epidemic was the bubonic plague or not, the bubonic plague returned in more localized outbreaks throughout the subsequent century. It struck England in 1665–1666, described by Defoe (1911) in his journal. There were varied epidemics in the Mediterranean countries and in Asia, including a serious outbreak in China in 1894. It even caused a scare when it appeared in San Francisco's Chinatown in 1907.

The disease that at least once, perhaps twice or even more, shattered humankind, seems far less virulent now. Modern medicine has reduced the mortality rate to less than 10%, which was once the rate of survival. It is likely that the infecting bacteria evolved into a milder form. This is to be expected. Evolution favors strains that do not rapidly kill their hosts. Then, too, in the developed world, changes in transportation, housing, and lifestyle have reduced exposure to the rat–flea–human cycle typified by the plague. Unlike their earlier counterparts, people today no longer consider flea infestation a normal part of daily life. The emergence of the brown rat over the black rat, and the construction of stone and brick housing, mean that most humans no longer live in close proximity to rats. The brown rat, too, now tends to be infected by different fleas and is less prone to plague. New modes of transporting goods preclude the infestation typical of the overland routes by which our forebears traded.

Cholera

Although the bubonic plague ceased its scourge, at least in the West, other diseases captured that same sense of dread. Most certainly cholera did. Cholera is a bacterial infestation of the intestinal linings, causing continuous diarrhea, intermittent vomiting, and severe abdominal pain. If untreated, cholera can cause rapid death due to dehydration. Almost nonexistent now in the developed world, cholera, still common in developing nations, is caused by the bacterium *Vibrio cholera*, found in polluted waters or on raw fruit and vegetables. It is treated today with antibiotics. In most cases, victims are hospitalized and given fluids intravenously to prevent the rapid dehydration associated with the disease.

The current complacency about the disease, at least in the developed world, contrasts sharply with the sense of dread and devastation the disease provoked less than two centuries ago. As Rosenberg (1962) stated, "Cholera was the classic epidemic of the nineteenth century as Plague had been of the fourteenth" (p. 1). Cholera, too, seems an old disease. Marks and Beatty (1976) found some ambiguous references to cholera in India as early as 400 B.C., with other inferences around 1325 A.D. But he judges the first reliable reports identifying cholera, also from India, date it in 1768–1769.

Four major pandemics struck the world in rapid succession from 1817 through 1875, striking most sections of the world and killing perhaps as many as millions. Although the mortality rate was not as high as for other diseases (e.g., more Americans died of malaria or tuberculosis), it terrified the population because it was a new disease that both spread rapidly and killed quickly.

But it did not always strike all populations equally. As Dr. John Snow, a London physician, would show later in the pandemic, cholera existed where sanitation was poor. Hence the poor suffered disproportionately. And, as in AIDS, the victims were blamed for their fate.

The disease, which had been somewhat endemic in India, now spread to the rest of the world. Three things facilitated this movement. During this time, the British economic and military penetration of India provided opportunities for the disease to move beyond geographic boundaries. Sleek ships rather than plodding caravans could now rapidly spread the disease. Second, once the disease spread, it entered a world that was far more mobile. Migrations and movements of people hastened its spread. Moslem travelers spread it throughout the Moslem world when the disease struck during the 1831 pilgrimage to Mecca (McNeill, 1976) and Irish immigrants brought it to the New World. Third, cholera struck at a time of rapid industrialization and urbanization throughout the world. Public sanitation, water, and sewer systems were nonexistent in many urban areas. This gave ample opportunity for the bacteria to spread.

Because the disease disproportionately struck the poor, it fanned class resentments and hatred. As with HIV, many of those infected with the disease, or at least those at risk, suspected the authorities of either developing the disease or facilitating its spread. In Poland and other parts of Eastern Europe, physicians, already poorly regarded by peasants, were suspected of poisoning the poor to kill off a surplus population. In Paris too, the poor saw the aristocracy as seeking to poison the poor. In the United States it was the poorer urban classes, particularly the Irish and Blacks, that suffered from the "poor man's plague." Although the Roman Catholic priesthood received some respect and sympathy for ministering to victims, the disease fanned an anti-Catholic and anti-immigrant prejudice that had been generated by the first mass migration of Catholics, who were seemingly prone to cholera. Cholera gave the Protestant majority one more reason to hate and fear the Catholic migrants.

The disease exacerbated the class conflicts. The suspicions and fears of the poor were sometimes confirmed in the attitudes of the upper classes. For example, the *Western Sunday School Messenger* drew a moral from the disease: "Drunkards and filthy, wicked people of all descriptions, are swept away in heaps, as if the Holy God could no longer bear their wickedness" (Rosenburg, 1962, p. 44).

Durey (1979) characterized the wealthier classes as having a threefold response to the crisis. First, they denied the existence of the disease because it affected commercial and shipping interests with threats of quarantine. Second, they had a sense of calm that the disease would serve to rid society of its most undesirable elements. In an age where ideas compatible to social Darwinism were beginning to be heard, some saw cholera as a "culling of the herd," echoes of which are still pronounced in some commentators' views of AIDS. Third, the wealthier classes also responded with fright and resentment of the poor when cholera began to spread through society at large.

In many ways the cholera pandemic raised the status of medicine, developed public health, and even rejoined medicine and society. As in earlier pandemics, there were different theories of disease. Some felt the disease was due to atmospheric conditions, local "miasmas," or unhealthy air that allowed diseases to flourish. Others held that diseases were complex interactions of atmospheric seasons and individual constitutions. Still others held that contagious pathogens spread disease. It was also a perspective that allowed actions—quarantines and sanitary cordons—to stem the disease. These actions were not always popular at the time. The wealthy resented the quarantines' effect on their commercial interests. The poor often believed sanitary cordons were designed so that they would be held in disease-ridden ghettos and kept from traveling. These actions signaled the beginnings of public health. Cholera also affirmed the relationship between social conditions and health, shaking, in the West, a sense of superiority over what were perceived as less civilized sections of the world.

Although cholera struck at a time when science was ascendant, theological explanations of the disease still existed, as they exist for AIDS today. To some, cholera was a divine punishment of the afflicted. To others, it was a judgment on a society that tolerated slums and poverty.

Typhus and Typhoid Fever

Improved sanitation and health measures eased the threat of cholera in Europe and America. But other epidemic diseases recaptured that sense of dread. Similar to cholera, typhoid fever is caused by the bacillus *Salmonella typhosa*, found in human feces and spread by contaminated food and water. Again, typhoid fever is characterized by symptoms similar to those of cholera—diarrhea, abdominal discomfort, as well as fever. Typhus, spread by body lice, as is the plague, is evidenced by high fever, violent headaches, and rash.

Although typhus and typhoid fever are quite dissimilar, both thrive in unsanitary conditions. Both often have followed in the wake of wars. Zinsser (1934), in his classic work, *Rats, Lice and History*, argued that typhus changed the course of history numerous times, often tipping the scales in critical battles. It is rats and lice, and perhaps the sanitation officers who tried to control them, that affected history, Zinsser concluded, rather than the generals credited with the victory.

A similar case could be made for typhoid. Like typhus, it too was a factor on the battlefield, critically weakening armies. In wars, people more often died of typhoid than from combat.

Typhoid also contributed one character to history unrivaled, until perhaps Gaetan Dugas, the "patient zero" who Shilts (1987) believed contributed so much to the early spread of HIV. Mary Mallon, or "Typhoid Mary," was an uninfected carrier of the typhoid bacillus. From a position as an itinerant cook, she infected hundreds with the disease and continued her profession even after an initial quarantine until she was quarantined for a second and final time in New York City's isolated North Brother Island.

Although typhoid and typhus never captured the dread that outbreaks of cholera and bubonic plague did, they did engender more localized panic and turmoil, particularly in Eastern Europe in the tempestuous era following World War I, where more than three million persons died from typhus. There the diagnosis of typhus would demoralize a population already facing other horses of the apocalypse—famine and war. Eastern Europe was particularly susceptible after World War I. Whatever stability had existed had been broken by the Russian revolution and the breakup of the Austrian–Hungarian Empire. Without the major powers to enforce a tenuous peace, and with the rising tide of revolution and counteractions, Eastern Europe was in a constant state of turmoil between civil wars and wars between new nations eager to expand their boundaries and power.

The Influenza Epidemic

Perhaps one reason that the major European epidemic of typhus did not engender the same sense of dread as cholera was that a virulent strain of an old[2] and common disease had surpassed typhus and typhoid as a major threat, creating its own panic. Influenza is a disease that most people experience intermittently throughout their lives. Most of the time, unless one is weakened by infirmity or age, it is not life-threatening, just inconvenient. In fact, these separate outbreaks are actually caused by different, albeit related, viruses.

The influenza virus is extremely adaptable or mutable. Most changes are minor, called antigen drift. These changes still allow at least a partial defense from the immune system of people already infected with a prior variant of the virus, limiting the disease's effect. Sometimes, however, the changes are more significant and represent major genetic reassortment, called an antigen shift. It is these shifts that tend to produce the major pandemic of the disease, such as the Asian flu of 1957 or the Hong Kong flu of 1969. These shifts may occur from a variety of sources—virus mutation, adaptation of an animal virus to humans, or hybridization between a human and animal strain (Beveridge, 1977). With integrated farming more common now (e.g., raising swine, ducks, and chickens together) in Asia, the traditional birthplace of the flu, some suggest that influenza shifts may become more common as related influenza viruses of these animals have opportunities to commingle and to develop new mutations that can affect humans. Pandemics may become increasingly common as well.

It was one of these antigen shifts that produced the virus responsible for the misnamed Spanish flu of 1918–1919 that also probably originated in Asia. No one really knows why this particular variant was so deadly. Some suggest that there may have been co-features such as Pfeiffer's bacilli that contributed to the death toll (Crosby, 1977).

But it was deadly. The mortality rate from the disease was comparatively low, estimated from about 0.5 to 3% (Beveridge, 1977; Crosby, 1977). However, because close to 20% or more of the population contracted the disease, it is estimated that the death toll ranged between 21 and 37 million people. Here again, the mobilization of millions of soldiers in less than sanitary conditions provided a rich field for the virus to spread.

[2]Hippocrates reports an influenza epidemic as early as 412 B.C. A major pandemic occurred in 1510. Neither had the mortality rates of this epidemic (Beveridge, 1977).

Death was often quick. Stories abounded of persons riding to work well but never returning home. These stories still cast a shadow even to children who grew up in the 1950s. One old house I avoided as a child was said to be haunted. A young wife was quarantined there with influenza. Her husband took ill at work and later died in a hospital. She was said to have died alone at home, waiting for her husband to return and care for her, unknown in her new community. Younger adults, especially those in the close quarters of the military, were particularly vulnerable. The mortality rate also differed by areas. Some areas, such as the South Pacific, were particularly devastated.

The pandemic disappeared almost as quickly as it came. The third wave of the disease in the spring of 1919 was milder. Some suggest that the virus produced a variant that now infects swine.

In its brief history, however, influenza has created a deep sense of dread. As with cholera, it was a humbling experience, reminding science and the populace that epidemic diseases were not simply past scourges. It also demonstrated that medical science, despite its progress, was limited in the face of such a massive epidemic. It heightened tensions in nations still at war with Germany and in conflict with themselves over race. And it again raised issues of public health mandates versus individual freedom over such questions as quarantines and mandatory face masks.

DISEASE AND SOCIETY

The Effects of Epidemics

It is easy to understand the fear that these great plagues generated. Every individual was at risk. Persons legitimately feared not only for themselves but also for their progeny. Families and surnames were wiped out. Whole communities vanished. For the survivors, life was irrevocably changed. Fortunes were made and broken.

Even institutions, such as religion, changed. McNeill (1976) saw the early epidemics facilitate the growth of Christianity, because the Christian duty to care for the sick brought the new faith both visibility and commendation. Epidemics may have affected the relative power of religion in other ways as well. As mentioned earlier, the plagues may have set the stage for the Protestant Reformation by gripping the Roman Catholic Church in a judgmental theology that lasted far beyond the plague. McNeill also suggested that Islamic fatalism often mitigated against aggressive responses to diseases, such as quarantine. He proposed that this may have affected Mongol power and changed the demographic pattern in the Balkans where growing Christian majorities would later lead liberation movements against the Moslem Ottoman Empire. In any case, it is clear that religious customs can either facilitate or slow the spread of disease. And the presence of disease may well affect religious customs. In many Christian church bodies, for example, the specter of AIDS has led to modifications of rituals, such as moving toward alternatives to a common cup for communion.

Humans suffer from a peculiar form of "species-ism" that makes us reluctant to see microbes as central players in the course of human history. We like to believe that human destiny is in human hands. But these plagues often were turning points—some large, others small.

The major effects are still debated. Some see the bubonic plague as responsible for the decline of feudalism and the Islamic empire (e.g., Bowsky, 1978; Claster, 1982; Hourani, 1991). But beyond these major turning points these epidemics are full of stories that show wide-ranging, spidery effects. For example, Albert Fall, later a major player in the U.S. Teapot Dome Scandal, owed his close election to the sympathy generated by the loss of his two children in the influenza epidemic. Winning by less than 2,000 votes, Fall's election gave the GOP the Senate, setting the stage for the defeat of Wilson's League of Nations. The cemetery movements that sought to move graves out of churchyards into large park-like tracts received impetus from the influenza epidemics. It was often thought the graveyards contributed to the disease. There were financial effects as well. The fledgling insurance industry was almost overwhelmed by the death of so many young persons during the influenza epidemic. In small ways and great ones this disease altered human life.

They were also mirrors to life. More than historical turning points the epidemics were social mirrors, forcing societies to view the ways they responded to crises. As such, they forced society to face the limits of scientific theory and technology. The diseases also exposed the fault lines and tensions of the societies they struck.

Understanding Disease: The Limits of Science

In many ways, the different scientific explanations of successive epidemics illustrate the development of scientific thought. The rudimentary beginnings of medical science, based on Roman and Greek thought, had been overwhelmed by the plague of Justinian. Unable to explain or stem the epidemic, they sought alternative theological explanations.

During the Black Death, scientific accounts varied little from lay explanations. What passed for science was often a bad mix of religion, pseudosciences, and perhaps the very beginnings of scientific observations.

Some learned men of the time emphasized astrological explanations, blaming the plague on the triple concoction of Mars, Jupiter, and Saturn. Other scholars thought the atmosphere was to blame. They believed the air was fouled by noxious fumes released from earthquakes and volcanoes, or mounds of Eastern unburied dead, or by an evil mist drawn up of poisoned waters from the Indian Sea, which had been corrupted by massive fish kills. They credited unusual geographic conditions and weather with a sense that the earth itself had been wounded (Hecker, 1840/1846). Still others began to develop a contagion theory, that is, that the disease was contracted by contact with the bedding, clothes, or the person of those infected. It was these very early, undeveloped theories of contagion that led to the beginnings of public health measures and policies, mostly expressed in quarantines. The term "quarantine" was named after a policy in some Italian port cities that made ships wait 40 days before crews and/or goods embarked.

Some of these theories would resurface in subsequent epidemics, particularly the cholera pandemics, where the debate would rage between scientists who were "contagionists"—those who thought the disease could be spread, by some mechanism, from person to person—and "anticontagionists." The most popular anticontagionist theory was an environmental one. Like earlier theories, this one blamed a "miasma" or a foulness of the air and atmosphere for the disease.

The debate between the proponents of these theories was often bitter and many times spilled over into severe disagreements over public health policy. Anticontagionists often saw little reason to support quarantines and sanitary cordons. There were, however, some areas of public health that they could commonly support even if for very different reasons. Sanitation, for example, was generally supported by both; contagionists saw mounds of garbage and untreated sewage as breeding grounds for infection and anticontagionists believed it fouled the atmosphere. Similarly, the cemetery reform movement's goal to develop cemeteries outside of overcrowded churchyards in the city center was supported by both groups.

The cholera epidemic represents a turning point in many ways for modern science. Dr. Snow's detective work traced the source of the epidemic to an infected well. His discovery of this infected well brought prestige to the medical community and success to the contagionists, a success that would be triumphant with subsequent medical discoveries. Throughout the cholera epidemic the status of doctors rose. In the early 1800s physicians were poorly regarded. Hospital mortality was high and, in some countries, such as Britain, there had been inflammatory scandals that besmirched the medical profession. For example, two Englishmen, Burke and Harre, had murdered 18 people and sold the bodies to a medical school. This introduced a new slang word into the British vocabulary, "burked" (referring to being killed and having one's body sold as medical supply) and a new fear, especially among the poor, that a visit to the hospital could lead to a "burking." The epidemic did, however, force physicians into the public eye. In the absence or inaction of public health boards, it was often medical societies that took an active role in organizing responses to the threat posed by the epidemic.

If these epidemics demonstrate the emergence of science, they also show its limits. At its very best, medical science could answer the "how" questions—how a disease could develop and spread. But it could not answer the "who" question. From the very first, overseers noted that some people would contract disease, whereas others would not. Some would succumb to death but others would survive. Contagionists could neither predict nor explain why any given individual contracted a disease and died. The explanations echo today—individual proclivity, lifestyle, mystery, luck, God's punishment. And science could not answer the "why" questions: Why has this disease occurred now? Why was this flu so deadly? Why did so many die? In fact, in the more recent epidemics, especially that of influenza, the inability of science to control the disease stunned a population that had considered such plagues a relic of the past.

In addition to scientific attempts to understand and master disease, there were lay understandings and responses to the disease. Two of the more popular were, then and now, denial and avoidance. Denial often took on characteristic forms: "The disease will not reach here, or if it does it will not touch my strata or group." Often there were strong commercial undertones to denial of an epidemic that would radically affect trade and economic life. Cholera provides an effective illustration of denial, especially in America. As Americans heard of the migration of the disease into Europe, they still assumed that the disease would stop at the Atlantic. Even when the disease appeared in Canada in June 1832, Americans, believing they were free of the poverty and degradation associated with Europe, felt that the disease would not have a great effect on them. Once it did strike, first infecting a few Irish migrants in New York City at the end of June 1932, many still hoped and assumed that the disease would stay within the city, the slums, the Irish, and the poor. Cholera was still considered a consequence of predisposing factors—immoral, intemperate, or filthy lives. Although different groups believed cholera was a consequence of sin, bad social conditions, or simply lack of sanitation, the implication was that clean living, whether that meant church going or healthy lifestyles, would protect one from risk.

Cholera illustrated, too, the economic press for denial. In both the United States and Europe, commercial interests often conflicted with physicians— initially over diagnosis, then over policy. The scare of cholera meant ships from the area were likely to be quarantined. Sanitary cordons affected inland codes of health. Because boards of health were more vulnerable to economic and political pressures, medical societies often became instruments for physicians to struggle against the emerging epidemics, sometimes finding themselves accused of usurping the role of the pliant health boards.

When denial was no longer possible, avoidance became a customary response. Avoidance took a number of forms. When possible, people fled from the disease, often spreading the disease as they traveled. Frequently, this flight had class connotations, for only the wealthier classes had the leisure to travel and places to go, such as country homes.

If one could not leave, one could at least avoid those infected. The fear of disease many times fragmented social order. Winslow (1943), for example, quotes one witness to the Black Death: "A father who did not visit his son, nor the son his father. Charity was dead! . . . Even the doctors dare not visit the sick from fear of infection" (p. 98).

This avoidance was often reflected in policies. Cities and countries closed borders or quarantined parts to restrict entry. Quarantines began in the eras, especially during the time of the Black Death, when there was little scientific support or justification for them. They simply expressed a collective will both to avoid and to do something in the face of the terror of death. These actions were acceptable as long as they affected others. When they threatened one's own movement or interests, they were bitterly divisible.

Blame and Disease

There was also a more ominous response to the disease—that of scapegoating others. The failure of science to explain why the disease had erupted led persons to blame others. Surely, they reasoned, if not for the active intervention of some enemy, this disease could not randomly and suddenly appear. Sometimes the enemy was external. The influenza epidemic was popularly blamed on the Axis powers, especially Germany. The assumption was (despite the fact that Germans were dying from the disease) that the Germans directly caused this plague, releasing infection from U-boats and spoiled medicines and indirectly as a result of poison gas. The suspicions and rumors were such that the U.S. Public Health Service was forced to test the purity of Bayer aspirins, because the company had German roots. Similarly, Catholic Spanish Christians had accused the Moslem King of Grenada of spreading the Black Death. Interestingly enough, this has been repeated with HIV; in the 1980s the KGB circulated accounts that AIDS had been manufactured by the CIA as an exercise in biowarfare.

Along with external enemies, internal groups were often blamed for the disease as well. In some cases it was believed that these groups acted at the request of external enemies. For example, the Moslem King of Grenada was accused of using lepers and Jews to spread the plague. In other cases these groups were simply believed to spread the plague as an act of vindictiveness. For example, lepers and cripples were accused of spreading the disease so others might share the misery and isolation. As Guy de Chaulie, a witness of the plague, wrote: "In some cases they believed it was the Jews that poisoned the world, so they killed them. In other places, they believed it was the poor cripples, so they drove them away" (quoted in Winslow, 1943, p. 98).

During the Black Death, Jews were often accused of poisoning wells and spreading the plague. Ziegler (1969) suggested that the pervasive rumors of well poisoning were rooted in the Jewish custom, born of the sanitary practices and laws as well as communal restrictions, of drawing water from open streams rather than village wells. These rumors, which seemed to begin in 1348 in Chillan (Marks & Beatty, 1976), were readily believed in societies characterized by a persistent anti-Semitism and suspicions that Jews were responsible for hosts of evils such as sacrificing Christian children. Furthermore, the deep theological underpinnings of the plague, the popular understanding that the plague was punishment for sins, provided a context in which tolerance of heresy and unbelievers was as responsible for the plague as poison. Persecutions of the Jews were also fanned by torture and trials that forced confessions and by the Flagellants, a religious movement, who in their processions whipped up anti-Semitic passions. Despite the attempted interventions of rulers like the Emperor Charles IV and Pope Clement VI's pleas that Jews were just as much victims of the plague as anyone, the pogroms forced many Jews to migrate to the East. Tuchman (1978) saw the plague beginning the isolation of the Jews in certain areas, which would later develop into full ghettos. Between the plague, persecutions, and migrations, many Jewish communities in Europe disappeared (Ziegler, 1969). Although the Jews were the most common scapegoats of the plague, they were not the only ones. Other marginalized groups such as homosexuals, heretics, lepers, and cripples were also blamed for the deaths. Again, much of the same patterns are seen with the AIDS epidemic, as each group sees another group as responsible.

Many reactions to these great epidemics were transcendental. Given the religious interpretations of the disease, this is not surprising. Religious conversions and renewed devotions were not uncommon. During the cholera epidemic there were calls for a national day of fasting and repentance. Again, it was the Black Death that generated an intense religious movement called the Flagellants.

The Flagellants, officially the Brothers of the Cross, began in Central Europe in the 1340s. The movement originally began as a collective attempt at repentance to assuage God's evident wrath. The Flagellants moved in elaborate processions from town to town. Although the groups were usually between 200 and 300, they sometimes numbered more than 1,000. It was a fearsome and gloomy show. The men, headed by a master, would march in the front, women in the rear. Their faces in cowls, their eyes on the ground, they would be silent except for hymns. Members swore to scourge themselves at least three times a day, for 33 days and 8 hours (representing Christ's life). Because their rules prohibited bathing, Ziegler (1969) concluded that some of this scourging had to be ritualistic, or else they would die of infection.

As time and plague continued, the Flagellants became more extreme. As stated earlier, they often encouraged anti-Jewish pogroms. Under increasing suspicion by the church, they became increasingly anticlerical. They also began to become chiliastic, believing their movement would, after 33 years, bring on Christ's final judgment. Tolerated initially by the church, their theology and behaviors finally led to condemnation by a papal bull in 1349 and complete suppression by 1457 (Tuchman, 1978).

Responses in Literature and Art

Another typical response to these epidemics was expression in humor, song, and story. Few probably remember the 1918 jumping rope chant:

> I had a little bird its name was Enza.
> I opened the window and in-flew-Enza.

Most of us, however, sang "Ring Around the Rosie" as children, oblivious to its roots as a chant to ward off disease. Few realize that the story of the Pied Piper was a thinly veiled allegory to the bubonic plague, with the Pied Piper, symbolizing in his multicolored clothing the discolored skin of victims, taking away both rats and children. The HIV epidemic too has spawned all forms of literary responses, from serious drama [e.g., *Angels in America* (Kushner, 1993), etc.] to gentle movie comedy (e.g., *Jeffrey*) as well as expressions in art, dance, other fiction, and nonfiction. It has also generated a body of humor that ranges from the cruel to the ironic and touching.

The middle ages especially spawned a macabre form of art that personified death. Fulton and Owen (1988) suggested that perhaps because the dead were buried so rapidly, without much ritual, death became fascinating, even erotic. It also generated an unusual form of literature, the ars moriendi (or artes moriendi), which means "the art of dying." These books were guides for those preparing to die as well as those that might minister to them. The ars moriendi, while describing the temptations of life and the horrors of dying, also provided comfort that one could survive the crisis of death and make a transition to heaven.

All of these responses, Kastenbaum and Aisenberg (1976) suggested, offered an emotional counterattack to epidemic death. It gave a society that technologically, medically, and even socially could not cope with the massive death toll ways to do something, to recapture in some way a sense of control over disease and thereby lessen the unmitigated horror and devastation of death.

Responding to Disease: The Limits of Reason

These great epidemics exposed not only the limits of science, but the limits of reason. Individually, the range of responses varied from panic to resignation, hysteria to heroism. Collectively, the tensions of disease surfaced the basic conflicts that had simmered in those societies. Like an earthquake eroding fault lines, the epidemic tore apart the covers of societies, allowing prejudices and passions expression.

The religious conflicts were discussed earlier. The Black Death intensified the religious hatreds of the medieval world, pitting Christians against Jews and Moslems. Later epidemics also exposed other simmering religious tensions. The 1832 presidential campaign in the midst of the cholera epidemic raised issues related to the ongoing conflict in American society between the separation of church and state. President Andrew Jackson's refusal to proclaim a national day of fasting and repentance, citing separation of church and state, became a campaign issue intensely dividing orthodox Christians and radicals and exposing the anticlericalism of some of Jackson's supporters. The clamor continued for more than a decade until President Zachary Taylor finally recommended a day of fasting. The same cholera epidemic also surfaced resentment toward Roman Catholic migration to an overwhelmingly Protestant America. In the current ecumenical age, it seems hard to remember that anti-Catholicism once aroused extremely strong passions. But at the time migration to the Americas began, the religious wars between Protestants and Catholics had barely ended, and religious divisions were still major ideological rifts.[3] Even the influenza epidemic in 1919 caused religious controversies. The bans on public gatherings such as religious processions deeply offended the faithful and were opposed by some clergy.

The epidemic spurred racial and ethnic conflicts as well. For example, the influenza epidemic not only led to suspicions about Germans and, by extension, German Americans, it is cited as a contributory factor to the bloody racial riots in the summer of 1919. Race also figured in the U.S. outbreak of cholera. Again in the New York slums, African Americans suffered high death rates and faced the added stigma of disease. The last U.S. outbreak of the bubonic plague also showed racial fault lines. Anti-Asian prejudice had been evident in the Western states from the 1870s. When the plague first appeared in San Francisco's Chinatown, it was vigorously denied by some state officials and newspapers. But worried public health officials, supported by Hearst's newspaper, the *Examiner*, sought to mount a vigorous defense. The actions, however, in quarantining Chinatown and attempting to forcibly detain residents and restrict access of Asians to public transportation suggested racial discrimination. In fact, the latter two actions, supported by the U.S. Surgeon General, were declared illegal by the courts. Not just race or ethnicity, but any form of social marginality, made such groups collective targets of the larger society, a fact witnessed by cripples and lepers during the Black Death.

One of the major fault lines in any society is social class. Class conflicts were often exacerbated during epidemics. In most of these epidemics the poor suffered both earlier and disproportionately. Yet this did not protect them from being blamed for the disease. Upper classes assumed that the poor's association with the disease was not simply a result of the condition of poverty (i.e., poor nutrition, sanitation, and housing), but rather choices to lead a decadent life. Poverty was still in many places considered a moral choice rather than a social fact. Some

[3]In the 1960 U.S. presidential election, John F. Kennedy's Roman Catholic faith was still perceived as a campaign issue and a possible liability.

saw England's "poor laws," which limited the mobility of the poor, as arising from a concern to minimize contact with the diseased lower class (Slack, 1988). Cholera especially was considered a disease of vagabonds and tramps. Even responses to the disease increased the sense of alienation of the poor. For example, newspaper suggestions in the cholera epidemic to retreat to summer homes must have seemed insensitive to the poor. In the United States, many cities gave instructions and advice only in English, despite the fact that many poor immigrant groups did not speak the language.

The poor also noticed their propensity to disease and blamed the rich, both for the condition that led to disease and for callousness. As with AIDS, many who were infected believed that the wealthy had willfully caused the disease. This concept was not hard to accept when some upper-class spokesman described the disease as a necessary evil to rid society of undesirable groups. Many times in the history of epidemic disease, the poor attacked those richer. In the typhus epidemics, in Eastern Europe, mobs attacked nobles. In the cholera epidemic, quarantines against the poor caused riots in France, Poland, and Eastern Europe.

Disease also fed political passions. The cholera epidemic illustrates this well. Cholera, striking Western societies during the democratic reform movements of the early 19th century, was subsumed into the debate. In England, many radicals and liberals saw the threat of cholera, which, ironically, was first ignored by the upper classes as a "Tory Hoax" because it diverted the commercial class (deeply concerned over the effects of the disease on shipping), cost the lower class jobs, and drew interest away from reform (Durey, 1979). But conservatives also read their own message in the disease. In France, Carlist propaganda stressed that cholera followed the same paths as subversive ideas (Delaporte, 1986). Even theories of the disease and responses to the disease showed ideological bias. Conservatives tended to favor contagionist theories and were favorable to quarantines. Liberals tended toward anticontagionist theories because they stressed a common source of infection such as an atmosphere shared by all. In addition, anticontagionist theories allowed liberals to oppose the segregation and restricted freedoms that quarantines entailed while still allowing them to advocate urban reform.

Finally, the epidemics had moral dimensions. Those who resisted infection, or, at least, escaped death, seemed morally superior to those who succumbed. In short, these epidemic diseases stripped away veneers, exposing and exacerbating in a crisis of fear, death, and hopelessness whatever tensions existed in the societies the disease struck.

The disease also exposed another conflict, one that transcended the other—the ending conflict between the self and the collectivity. There is an inherent tension between the freedoms and rights of an individual and those of the society as a whole. In whatever era an epidemic struck, however rights in that place and time were defined, these rights were in a dynamic tension with the perceived rights of a society to do whatever it needed to protect itself.

The first popular responses to epidemics were quarantines and isolation. Although in retrospect these ideas were well ahead of scientific theory and medically sound, at the time they were simply an expression of panic. They were a ritual cleansing of the community, isolating those who had disease. This tension over rights would continue. The rights of Mary Mallon (Typhoid Mary) to earn a livelihood were subordinated to the rights of a community to protect itself from infection. These conflicts continued. In San Francisco, during the influenza epidemic, a major controversy erupted over a city ordinance requiring individuals to wear medical masks in public. As with any conflict, often the rights of *which individuals* becomes a critical issue. Those who have less social power and prestige may be less able to protect their individual rights against the claims of the collectivity. The San Francisco quarantine on Chinatown in 1905 may have been less acceptable had it been applied to another area, rather than a ghetto housing a despised minority. Even in the case of Typhoid Mary, one could question if the situation were reversed, that if it were not a poor Irish servant infecting wealthy employees, would Mary Mallon have been so vigorously segregated.

Many of these restrictive actions proved counterproductive. The widespread slaughter of dogs and cats reported by Defoe (1911) in his account of the plague facilitated the spread of diseased rats. Alaskan Governor Rigg's attempt to protect the state from influenza by refusing ships carrying victims to disembark inhibited the shipment of medical supplies when the disease eventually struck (Crosby, 1976).

The plague still, though, poses a threat. In 1994, a new version of the pneumonic plague affected Surat, India. Perhaps it will be an isolated episode, another example of the fragility of third world health and sanitation systems. Yet it serves as a reminder that many "vanquished diseases" are never truly conquered. They wait for opportunities to develop and spread. And if this outbreak truly is pneumonic plague and it is not contained this time, or perhaps, some future time, in a world of jet travel, a reemergence of the plague could make AIDS seem like child's play. And as new books, such as *The Hot Zone* (Preston, 1994) or *The Coming Plague* (Garrett, 1994), suggest other plagues such as the fatal Hantavirus, or equally fatal and virulent Ebola fever, always seem ready to emerge. At present the very virulence of these diseases has checked their spread. Yet, like HIV, these viruses, or yet undiscovered ones, could mutate in ways or develop in populations that would allow a wider dispersion of disease. These epidemics both old and new clearly show not only the limits of science, but the limits of human reason when forced to confront the terror of massive death.

CONCLUSION

According to Rosenberg (1989), epidemics are best understood as dramaturgical events. In Act One, the epidemic is slowly acknowledged as it imperceptibly begins. It threatens social order, risking panic and social dissolution. In Act Two society tries to manage and understand the seeming randomness of death, attempting to explain the death toll in light of prevailing theological, moral, medical, or social ideology. In Act Three, a social response is negotiated using varied policies and rituals. Finally, the epidemic slowly winds down. But as the tide recedes, it leaves considerable debris, not the least of which is a society radically changed by the encounter, reminded not only of the fragility of its order and the limits of science, but also the tenuous balance that exists between humans and their complex environment. As will be seen in later chapters, AIDS will cause the human species to confront its vulnerabilities as it, perhaps radically, modifies our present social order.

Chapter **2**

SHAME AND STIGMA

If it be a short and violent death we have no leisure to fear it;
if otherwise, I perceive that according as I engage myself in
sickness, I do naturally fall into some distant contempt of life.
Michael de Montaigne, 1533–1592

There is another category of dreaded disease. These are diseases that are dreaded not so much for the social destruction they entail, but rather for the individual devastation that the disease brings. It is not the rapidity by which communities are struck by contagion but the slowness with which individuals succumb to death. These would include, at given times in human history, diseases such as cancer, tuberculosis, syphilis, and leprosy. These diseases share the characteristics of being chronic, terminal, disfiguring, and debilitating.

These diseases are not generally feared for epidemic death tolls. Cancer is not contagious, and the others vary in the degree of contagiousness. Nor are they uniformly fatal. Even early in its history, not all forms of cancer were deadly. Tuberculosis too could be controlled, at times even cured. And although leprosy and syphilis were fatal at an early point in their histories, even then they took decades to kill.

It was not contagion or death that sparked such deep dread. Rather than death, it was the quality of life that provoked fear. While each disease had its own fearsome characteristics, all left a mark of shame and stigma on their victims.

25

This chapter begins by reviewing a little of the nature and history of these diseases as well as the distinct ways that victims were treated. Even more so than the epidemic diseases, these diseases were blamed on the victims. The disease, itself, was often perceived as evidence of some fault, some sin or weakness of the victim. Inevitably, the victims were seen as bringing the disease on themselves because of moral transgression, sexual indiscretion, faulty lifestyle, or weak physical or psychological constitution. Blamed for the disease, victims suffered silently in shame separated from society.

THE SHAMEFUL STIGMAS

Leprosy

The name "leprosy" has become a metaphor for loathsomeness. The term "leper" is now a synonym for an isolated, diseased outcast. The stigma of leprosy reaches far back in our history; even in Biblical times lepers were cast out of their communities, doomed to wander as the walking dead. This was no mere metaphor; in medieval culture there was a separation ritual, the separate leprosorum, which was similar to a burial ritual, even to the point of dirt being thrown on the leper's head. As Brody (1974) noted, one medieval monarch felt the ritual was unnecessarily symbolic and thus burned or buried lepers alive. Once outcast, lepers' treatment varied. Often considered socially dead, they were denied any rights. In the Middle Ages, sometimes they were confined to leprosariums or lazarettos. At other times they were forced to wander, begging from town to town. In a few cases, they were permitted to live at home, secluded. In some third world cultures, lepers retain their loathsomeness—spouses divorce them, they are banned from public transportation, physicians refuse to treat them. But in other countries the disease seems to provoke little fear or disgust.

Certainly the condition itself, leprosy or Hansen's disease, seems an unlikely candidate to arouse such fear. Leprosy has two main forms. One form, the tuberculoid form, results when the immune system responds against the invading bacilli, often leaving hard, nodular swellings in the skin and mucous membranes of the eyes, nose, and throat. In the lepromatous form, the disease continues to spread, causing the loss of sensation. In all forms, including a mixed form, visible lesions can be seen. Yet the disease is only mildly contagious. It is a difficult disease to transmit. Generally the incubation period is 5 years to as many as 20 years. It is generally transmitted only after prolonged skin-to-skin contact. Some even believe that a larger part of the population is immune to infection.

Why then did leprosy generate such fear? Gussow (1989) concluded that perhaps the uncertainty of this disease played some role. Even today leprosy has many uncertainties. Its symptoms mimic other diseases. The form and treatment of the disease is sometimes uncertain. The incubation period is unclear. Some people seem immune even after prolonged intimate contact whereas a few seem to be infected after comparatively brief exposure. Factors related to infection, such as the role of genetics, are not fully understood. Gussow (1989) also suggested that the diseases that are progressive, chronic, nonfatal, insidious, visible, associated with lower standards of living, and not epidemic (thus allowing only a few to bear the brunt of stigma) tend to generate fear.

It is also clear that the stigma the disease created ebbed and flowed over time. For example, when the disease returned with the Crusaders, the stigma of the disease had eased because it was perceived that Crusaders could not be so cursed. The disease then became an opportunity to show compassion. Later, in the United States, the disease was viewed as generating pity that could be garnered to support foreign charities and missions. At the same time, it was also perceived a sign of the inferiority of non-White races, whether African Americans or Asian migrants. Near the same time, Norwegians defined their own infected peasants as a situation now to be compassionately considered. Their earlier neglect was another charge against perceived Swedish indifference, that would now be corrected with independence. Clearly, the definition of the stigma changed as political and social conditions warranted.

Finally, Gussow (1989) noted the very tradition of leprosy creates a frame that continues to influence our perception of the disease—so much so that those suffering with the disease and their advocates eschew the names "leprosy" or "leper," promoting and preferring the more innocuous sounding "Hansen's disease."

Ironically there exist questions as to whether the contemporary Hansen's disease is even the medical or ancient disease of leprosy. Certainly the fears of the disease do not match the current reality of leprosy. Medieval writers saw leprosy as highly contagious, sometimes threatening even those downwind. Ancient and medieval descriptions of the disease are often unclear and nonspecific, reflecting both characteristic styles of writing[1] and the indistinct symptomatology of leprosy. Some medieval writers differentiated "leprosy of the Arabs,"

---

[1]Medieval writers tended to offer copious quotes from authorities rather than their own clinical observations.

perhaps the parasite disease elephantiasis, from the "leprosy of the Greeks." It is possible that the disease has evolved and changed over the years. It is also possible that the early descriptions of leprosy may refer to another skin disease entirely.

It is highly possible that these older descriptions of leprosy include the disease now identified as Hansen's disease as well as other, seemingly related infections. And despite the fear it generated it seems to have infected only small numbers of people, perhaps 20,000 or less at its peak in the 1200s. After the bubonic plague, the incidence of leprosy declined even further. There may be a number of reasons for that decline. Certainly the plague, and perhaps the populace, killed many carriers. Perhaps changes in clothing and custom, such as more wool and wood fuel, led to less huddling and bedding together and limited its spread. Then too, other diseases may have entered its niche. Wool provided opportunities for bedbugs and lice to spread other diseases. Pulmonary tuberculosis spread more efficiently than leprosy and seems to confer some immunity to that disease. Perhaps even the underlying bacillus may have adapted evolving into other diseases such as syphilis (McNeill, 1976). In any case, Hansen's disease, although it still generated fear, remained only a threat in Scandinavia as the plague eased.

Nonetheless, it is ironic that leprosy has left such a legacy of fear. In noting its virtual disappearance in Europe in the 1600s (until the later age of colonialism), Gussow (1989) suggested that for all the fear and commentary, it probably never was a major health threat. Although there are still new cases each year in the United States, and the disease still exists in some tropical areas, it is generally controllable. So even though the disease no longer generates fear, it is still a metaphor of loathsomeness for all the diseases we now label the leprosies of our time.

Syphilis

Whereas the identity of leprosy may be somewhat unclear, the origin of syphilis has been hotly debated. Some see the disease as an ancient one, in both the Old and New World, perhaps even identified with leprosy at times that mutated into an acute, fatal, and violent form in Europe in the late 15th century. The majority opinion has viewed syphilis as a disease that originated in the Americas and was inadvertently imported to Europe by Columbus's crew just as diphtheria, smallpox, and measles were accidentally being brought into the New World during the era of exploration. In both circumstances, these new diseases rapidly decimated populations that had little immunity to them.

What is not debated is that a form of syphilis appeared during French King Charles VIII's siege of Naples in 1495. It quickly spread through Europe as young mercenary soldiers and accompanying camp followers, clearly a high-risk population, returned home. It was at this point, whatever its origin,[2] that syphilis was now clearly recognized. Whether or not the disease had been previously present in Europe, the tempestuous conditions of war and the increase in promiscuous behavior provided effective channels for the disease to spread.

It was still debated as to why and how the disease was spread. Theories of transmission were not well understood, although some observers did hypothesize a venereal transmission. The disease was blamed on a common variety of things—heresy, blasphemy, and licentiousness; the conjunction of the planets; and of course one another. The French blamed Naples; Naples blamed the French. Almost everyone in Europe blamed the Moors and the Turks. Every once in a while the Beghards (or holy beggars),[3] a mystic erotic and communal sect that roamed Europe, was blamed. Some blamed prostitutes; during the siege of Naples they were eventually expelled for spreading syphilis.

Syphilis is, of course, a venereal disease. That label is interesting because one rarely classifies diseases through their mode of transmission. Even the newer characterization of STD (sexually transmitted diseases) maintains that distinction and accompanying stigma. Syphilis, caused by the bacterium *Treponema pallidum*, has three stages. In the first stage painless ulcers are evident. In the second stage, the victim feels unwell and experiences swollen glands and a rash. In the third stage, the disease can be latent for years, but can flare up causing blindness,

[2]Lasagna (1975) reviewed the evidence for a New World hypothesis and noted that there were no descriptions of the disease prior to Columbus; many observers noted it was new and some blamed it on Columbus; the severity of this disease course suggests little immunity; and there is some evidence of the disease in North and South America prior to Columbus, though not in Europe. Contrary evidence suggests that there is some evidence of syphilis in China and perhaps Europe, though it is hard to authenticate the evidence. Saracen's ointment, which Crusaders used to treat leprosy, contained mercury, which would do nothing for leprosy but would work on syphilis; and it is hard to see how the disease spread so fast from such a small, returned fleet. In addition, Rosenbury (1971) believed that syphilis' relationship to two common tropical diseases, yaws and pinta, suggests that the disease evolved from these and spread to Europe.
[3]The group was actually named the Brethren of the Free Spirit. Believing God to be in each of them, they felt exempt from ordinary morality. They encouraged nudity, group sex, and free love, among other offenses to medieval morality.

insanity, paralysis, and other effects. It is the first two stages that are highly infectious.

This disease changed society in many ways, some immediately apparent, some subtle and still debated. Again, because medical science was of little immediate help, there was a return to religion. In an age that celebrated amorous adventure, chastity, even celibacy, found new support. Promiscuity declined as monogamy became more common. Altman (1986) credited syphilis as being a significant factor that led to the rise of Puritanism in England, a movement that had a significant role in the development of the United States. Waxed linen condoms became popular.

Other impacts were more subtle. Syphilis affected a variety of historical figures including explorers, writers, royalty, and national leaders. Among those in the latter categories were Henry VIII, Peter the Great, and perhaps even Adolph Hitler. Who can determine the ways that this bacterium influenced history through those it infected and how it affected the quality of life?

Like so many dreaded diseases, the treatment was often as difficult as the disease. At first victims were driven to leprosariums, here often even avoided by the lepers. Later many cities segregated them in pox houses. Because physicians had little to offer, or any desire to do so, many turned to barbers and self-proclaimed specialists. Ironically over time these so-called specialists developed treatment based on the use of mercury for varied skin diseases. Although it sometimes did offer a cure, some succumbed to mercury poisoning.

Eventually the disease became less virulent, but remained a persistent problem, always alive in consciousness. Many of the debates that currently surround AIDS—confidentiality, contact tracing, premarital or mandatory testing—had their origins in debates about syphilis. Similar fears were evident—that casual contact, even drinking from a common cup, could spread the disease or that it was deliberately spread by some of those infected. Indeed, syphilis becomes the first disease that creates a conflict, explored later in this chapter, between morality and secular rationalism that would bedevil treatment. In the end it was penicillin that removed the sense of dread. At a dramatic 1943 meeting of the American Public Health Association, Dr. E. M. Mahoney announced that penicillin had been found to be an effective treatment for syphilis. Although the effectiveness of penicillin lifted that deep sense of dread that followed syphilis, lessening the stigma of the disease, syphilis still retains a curious ambiguity. To some, especially males, it is an inconvenient badge of proud and riotous promiscuity, a mark of sexual conquest and machismo. But it still retains some silent unsavory stigma, a residue of earlier times.

Tuberculosis

It is only recently and in association with AIDS that tuberculosis (TB) has reemerged as a potential threat to health.[4] For until recently, at least in the developed West, only the tuberculin test was a reminder of a once, and perhaps now again, dreaded scourge.

But for much of history, tuberculosis (also known as consumption, the White Death, or White Plague) was a major killer. Like many of the dreaded diseases in this section, tuberculosis is an ancient disease. As far back as 5000 B.C., the disease is evident, and seemingly worldwide. Evidence of cases and descriptions of the disease are found throughout the early history of the world.

Caused by a bacteria that is transmitted in the septum of infected persons or through milk of cattle, the disease has a number of phases. In the primary phase, the invading bacteria is resisted by the immune system. In some cases the bacteria, unable to be destroyed, is walled in by fibrous capsules. In such cases, the disease can flare again whenever the defenses are weakened. In the second phase, the walled-in areas, often found in the lungs, reduce the ability to breathe, and gradually waste the person away.

Although tuberculosis is an ancient disease, it became widely known and feared in the 19th century. There are two reasons for the increased visibility. First, for much of its earlier history, tuberculosis was easily confused with other wasting diseases affecting the lungs such as silicosis and cancer. Second, the industrial revolution provided an environment conducive to the spread of the disease. The tuberculosis bacilli can survive in the droplets of cough for hours, lingering in the air. Overcrowded factories, tenements, and cities offered an ideal environment for the spread that was lacking in a more rural agrarian society.

Like AIDS, tuberculosis produced tremendous fear. It was unpredictable, for although the bacterium usually affected the lungs, it could affect any organ, producing diverse symptoms. In its time it was fatal, contagious, incurable, and had a long uncertain period of incubation. Its early symptoms (fever, weight loss, fatigue, a dry cough) were indistinct, mimicking many common conditions. As one survivor recalls:

[4]The interrelationship between AIDS and tuberculosis is indeed ominous. The current tests screening for tuberculosis can often come out negative because a diminished immune system may not provoke positive response on a tuberculin test even if the person tested is infected. This will facilitate the spread of the disease.

> In those days the specter of tuberculosis was as terrifying as
> cancer is today. Every third person between the ages of fifteen
> and sixty in the country—or about one in ten—died of TB. It
> was widely known to kill and, prior to death, to disable its vic-
> tims and reduce them to a state of helplessness. It was a wast-
> ing disease that was also highly contagious, which meant that
> sufferers were usually ostracized. (Mooney, 1979, p. 24)

The cause was debated for a considerable amount of time. Given that tuberculosis often spread through families, heredity was often considered at least as a
predisposing factor. Some others thought certain body types, particularly those
who were fair or tall, were particularly susceptible to the disease. The environment
of overcrowded cities was seen as dangerous. In fact, as Rothman (1994) indicates, it was this growing identification with the urban poor at the turn of the
century that was increasingly responsible for a growing stigmatization of the
disease. As TB first emerged in the early 19th century, it was greatly feared. But
at that point the disease seemed democratic. Anyone could get it. By the close of
the century it was considered a mark of shame, a reminder of dark tenements and
unsanitary conditions. Gradually contagion was suspected, and finally proved by
Koch in 1882 (Musto, 1988).

Finding the cause did little to effect an immediate cure. In fact, the triumph of
the contagion theory added further justification for the now growing ostracism
tubercular patients faced. Those who suffered from the disease were often housed
far from their habitats and occupations. Even hospitals and physicians refused to
treat them. In many areas it ended any marriage possibilities. Suspected TB
victims were often sorely discriminated against—removed from public transportation and markets. Although many famous persons succumbed including Saint
Bernadette, Frederick Chopin, Franz Kafka, and Henry David Thoreau, and although it did offer images of the romantic young woman wasting away, it was
primarily considered a disease of the poor, again a mark of poverty. In many
cases, doctors omitted this cause of death from the death certificate to avoid
stigmatizing survivors.

Like those of many dreaded diseases, victims of TB were often segregated
in sanatoriums. These sanatoriums, often placed in remote dry climates far
from a populace, offered a "rest cure." The remoteness of the sanatorium had
little to do with restfulness. Rather it reflected the resistance of communities
to having sanatoriums near them. In the late 1800s and early 1900s, rest in a
sanatorium and the radical therapy of collapsing a lung was the only available
treatment.

Over time tuberculosis became controlled. Although initially resisted by physicians as a violation of the doctor–patient confidentiality, many areas required physicians to report cases of the disease, allowing nascent public health organizations some means of control. Tuberculin tests, public education, the inspection of cattle, the pasteurization of milk, and the development of antibiotics gradually lessened the prevalence of TB in the Western world.

That is until recently. Now the AIDS epidemic, the rise of homelessness, and drug addiction provide reservoirs of persons with weakened immune systems that may allow a once fearsome scourge to return again and regenerate fear of the disease.

Cancer

Cancer is really not one disease but a series of different diseases each caused by uncontrolled cell growth. Again like many of these stigmatic diseases, cancer is an ancient illness. The earliest references to cancer are found in the Egyptian Eber's Papyrus (c. 1500 B.C.). It was Hippocrates who gave cancer its name, linking it to a crab perhaps because of the crab-like appearance of some tumors and similarity of the pain to the bite of the crabs, or its tenacious ability to spread.

Although cancer was recognized very early, there was considerable theorizing about the cause. Galen believed cancer occurred when black bile entered an area that was overexercised or injured. Others believed an imbalance of humors caused the disease. Others recognized environmental influences. Already in the 18th century, physicians had noted that persons who used snuff were at risk for developing nasal tumors, and that scrotal cancer seemed an occupational hazard for chimney sweeps. Others felt cancer was contagious, initiating a sense of horror and dread that would trouble victims. Still others believed cancer was hereditary; a notion that also contributed to a sense of shame and silence because it made family members less desirable as potential marriage partners. In 1926, Johannes Fibirger won the Nobel prize for a now discredited theory that cancer was a parasitic disease caused by nematode worms (Olson, 1989). Gradually though, in the 19th and 20th centuries, both the cell and germ theories, becoming widely accepted, led to the increasing recognition of a more modern theory of cancer. A German scientist, Rudolf Virchow, was instrumental in showing that cancer was a local, cellular disorder, with its own history, that seemed influenced by both heredity and environment.

Treatment too was comparatively late in developing. In early times surgical removal of the tumor was often attempted. Wilhelm Roentgen's discovery of x-rays at the turn of the century quickly became utilized as a new modality to treat cancer. In the 1940s chemotherapy also began to be applied as a third instrument of cancer treatment.

But with these medically accepted treatments, there always existed a strong cancer counterculture. In effect the comparative inability of medicine, especially early medicine, to treat cancer encouraged all forms of quackery or alternative approaches. Some of these even received considerable attention and credibility. The minutes of Virginia's House of Burgesses in 1748, for example, notes an award to a Mary Johns for a cure for cancer that consisted of garden sorrel, celandine, persimmon bark, and water (Olson, 1989).

Though cancer's history is ancient, the fear that it aroused did not emerge until the end of the 19th century. Sometimes a well publicized illness or death brings a disease into public consciousness. For AIDS, the death of Rock Hudson and the diagnosis of HIV infection in Magic Johnson were pivotal events, searing the illness into public awareness. In cancer's case, it was the long illness and eventual death of former U.S. President Ulysses Grant. Here the press, overcoming an earlier reluctance to mention cancer, chronicled Grant's suffering in great melodramatic detail.

Grant's illness came at a point in time when the public was becoming increasingly aware of cancer. There were a number of reasons for that. Cancer was more likely to be recognized and diagnosed. The increase in life expectancy made more people at risk for the disease. Industrialization created more exposure to carcinogens. Thus even without underlying statistics, there was a perception that this disease was now growing, striking victims at random, bringing pain, disfigurement, suffering, and death in its wake. Unlike other dreaded diseases, cancer had the continued fear of reoccurrence.

Although other diseases such as tuberculosis initially caused fear, cancer began to be seen as a disease to be denied and avoided. The term "cancer" became buried in euphemisms. For example, obituaries until recently (because it might be misconstrued as AIDS) noted that an individual died of "a long illness." Often the clothes of the dead were burned or buried. Cancer hospitals developed because other hospitals were reluctant to take cancer patients or be stigmatized as a cancer clinic. Despite the opinion of medical science, a poll in 1939 found 41% of the population believed cancer was contagious (Patterson, 1987), reflecting both the tenacity of the fear and stigma of the disease and the underlying, lingering distrust of the medical establishment that still is a staple of the cancer counter-culture.

In some ways, both the fear of the disease and the belief it struck at random were beneficial. Often cancer groups like the American Society for Control of Cancer, founded in 1913 and renamed the American Cancer Society in 1944, utilized that fear to induce support. Clarence Cook Little, an early leader of the group, organized popular opinion by mobilizing women's clubs and the media to persuade the federal government to take an unprecedented leap into actively supporting cancer research in 1937. The advocacy of the groups not only created the National Cancer Institute, but maintained cancer research as the number one health priority, a position it still retains.

This unprecedented federal role in supporting research was made possible for four reasons. First, the New Deal administration of Franklin D. Roosevelt had a vision of an activist role for the national government. Prior administrations would have been unlikely to perceive that the federal government had any legitimate role in sponsoring medical research. Second, the cancer advocacy groups, such as the American Cancer Society, were extraordinarily effective. They successfully managed a public relations and media campaign that emphasized that cancer was a growing health threat that placed anyone and everyone at risk. Their symbolism aptly avoided fragmenting the disease as a problem of any given group such as women or the poor. This gave everyone a sense of stake in the crusade. Third, the fear was tempered with optimism. Cancer is treatable, even curable. Efforts and funds then would not be perceived as wasted. Finally, the cancer lobby was reasonably unified. Except for the unorthodox researchers and adherents that still exist today, the cancer lobby was able to unite patient and family groups, major organizations, and the media in a common front. In fact their efforts opened the way for other groups and lobbies to press their own agendas; the cancer lobby became a model of success that other groups sought to emulate.

So although the American Cancer Society was accused of using cancer phobia to encourage research, it also promoted a sense of optimism. In the 1940s a survivor literature began to emerge recounting successful struggles of survivors. The moral of these stories was often twofold: first, that early detection and prompt treatment could lead to a cure, and second, that the wall of silence surrounding cancer had to be broken. If survivors emerged, it was reasoned, the shame and stigma of cancer would diminish, leading more to seek early treatment and therefore survive. In fact, as more persons have survived, and as the disease has become more open, cancer has emerged from its closet—leaving room for another dreaded disease, AIDS, to take its historical place.

Smallpox and Polio: On the Cusp

On the cusp of the two categories of dreaded diseases are smallpox and polio. Like the diseases discussed in the earlier chapter, both smallpox and polio were contagious and epidemic. Smallpox epidemics killed millions of people. Like many of the diseases described in this chapter, they were feared not only for their mortality but for the ways they disfigured and crippled survivors. In both cases, children were often victims.

Smallpox, so named to distinguish it from the great pox—syphilis—is caused by the variola virus. An acute disease, smallpox begins with a fever and then development of pus-filled lesions. Although, even in the early days, many, perhaps half, survived the disease, it left permanent scars that could sometimes grossly disfigure or even blind survivors. This disfigurement could take deep personal toll. In some cases, weddings were canceled and children abandoned.

The disease, too, seems ancient, evident in China and India as far back as the 11th century B.C. It seemed to enter the West with traders, perhaps first in Alexandria. Moslem invaders brought the disease into Spain in 210 A.D. Because the Spanish had no immunity, the disease was as devastating as the Muslim conquest. It would take the Spanish more than 700 years to reclaim their country from those invaders. Ironically, smallpox along with mumps and measles had the same effect when the Spanish invaded South America. There, too, the epidemics of smallpox, brought on by infected slaves, decimated the Aztecs and Incas, who had no natural immunity. Wracked by disease, and dispirited by the devastation of their society, Incan and Aztec cultures were soon overwhelmed by what was perceived as a superior European culture. It was not only the guns and horses of the Spanish but also their diseases that facilitated their conquest. These diseases too would have a similar role in North America. In North America the disease generally spread to North Americans as an inadvertent aspect of contact with Europeans. But sometimes it was not inadvertent. One British general, Sir Jeffrey Amherst, in 1763, practiced a form of biological warfare when he deliberately delivered smallpox-contaminated blankets to the Iroquois.

Smallpox was also one of the first diseases to be controlled. The story has become legendary. In 1796, an English country doctor, Edward Jenner, noticed that milkmaids who had developed a mild disease related to smallpox, called cowpox, did not seem to develop smallpox. Because it was known that smallpox conferred lasting immunity on survivors, Jenner reasoned that if he inoculated people with cowpox they would gain immunity from smallpox. Jenner's work inspired others. In perhaps the first significant public health campaign, the Spanish

King Carlos IV, after his daughter's recovery from smallpox, ordered the vaccination of all of Spanish America and the Philippines. Twenty-two young orphans were serially vaccinated with smallpox as they crossed the ocean so that fresh cowpox would be available to begin a chain of vaccination. It would take almost 200 years before worldwide vaccination campaigns would eradicate the disease. Eventually the viruses, eliminated from their hosts, lived in only two high-security laboratories as scientists debated both the wisdom and the ethics of destroying this once dreaded microbe. It was supposed to have been destroyed in 1995.

Like smallpox, polio was known as a disease of children. But whereas smallpox disfigured survivors, polio crippled. Poliomyelitis, or polio as it was shortened by news editors, seems to be an old disease. But although the disease can arguably be traced back as far as ancient Egypt, it is only in the last century that polio became more common and noticed.

Although many diseases like cholera were controlled through modern hygiene, polio seems to be an inadvertent byproduct of modern sanitation. The polio virus is widespread and ubiquitous in fecal manner. When infants were exposed to it early they generally suffered what passed for a minor cold, or perhaps as Paul (1977) suggested polio was just an unrecognized part of high child mortality rates. Later improved sanitation made it more epidemic than endemic. Although the first U.S. epidemic occurred in Vermont in 1894, others would follow in 1916 and the 1950s. In any case in the modern era, increased cleanliness meant that children were less likely to be exposed to the virus until later in life when its effects were more dangerous. For persons having no prior immunity, the disease could be more devastating. If the virus struck the central nervous system, death and paralysis could occur. In some cases, paralysis of the spinal cord meant the victim could only breathe with the help of the mechanical and dreaded "Iron Lung." In polio epidemics, probably most children were infected, and many had no or minor symptoms, but at least 2–4% suffered central nervous system involvement.

Despite the fact that more children died from accidents than polio, the disease still generated intense fear. For those who grew up in the 1950s, a series of images still stand. I remember Richard and Mary, two classmates who walked with frightening, clanging braces. I remember strangers telling us when we splashed in a puddle or played hard that we might get polio, and trips to beaches and pools were denied as attempts to limit exposure to the disease. Families that could, tended to flee infected cities, sometimes bringing disease with them. Hospitals often refused polio patients, particularly in the 1916 epidemic, leaving them isolated in special hospitals. Houses were quarantined and children under 16 were not permitted to leave without a certificate that they were polio free.

Again, theories of disease varied. Although the germ theory was clearly established by this time, other options were considered. Again in the first polio epidemic immorality was blamed for the emergence of this new threat. Because the children could scarcely be immoral, parents, particularly fathers, were blamed. The emergence of influenza in 1918, and other diseases in the 1920s such as encephalitis in Japan, the Australian X disease, and the encephalitis lethargica in Europe, led some researchers to wonder if some new factor had increased the susceptibility of the central nervous system to infection. Some researchers even attempted severing the olfactory nerve, believing polio could somehow be prevented by the loss of smell. Parents had their own ideas. During polio epidemics, many parents believed keeping their children bathed, rested, well fed, and away from crowds was the best protection. Schools and camps ceased to operate.

Three things gradually eased the fear. First, Franklin Roosevelt's presidency provided a positive role model of how polio could be surmounted, giving the disease a heroic cast. Second, the work of Sr. Kenny with polio victims in the 1940s generated great sympathy. Third, and most importantly, the Salk and Sabin vaccines eased the fear and gradually brought, at least in the developed world, polio under control. In a review of the history of polio, Paul (1971) speculated as to whether the decline of the polio virus will lead to other viruses within that common Coxsackie viral family emerging and infecting humans. At present, he concludes, this does not seem to have occurred.

BLAMING THE VICTIM: THE CONNOTATION OF DISEASE

Although the great epidemics generally aroused anger at outside enemies and marginalized groups within the afflicted society, stigmatized diseases were often blamed on the victim. There were three reasons for this. First, the great suffering that these diseases caused naturally led one to assume that in some way the victim must be responsible for his or her own fate, and is being punished for his or her sins. After all, unlike the great epidemic diseases, these diseases were comparatively selective in afflicting individuals; therefore it could be assumed that the individuals somehow must have merited the diseases.

Second, this thinking was protective. The anguish these diseases caused was obvious. It was terrifying to think that this was even somewhat random. On the other hand, if these diseases were a punishment, or in some way the fault of the individual afflicted, it restored hope that one could avoid that fate.

Third, as science progressed, it became clear that some of these diseases involved lifestyle issues. Certainly cancer did. Diet, occupation, and habits were identified early as factors that seemed to affect the chances of developing cancer. As early as the 18th century, an English surgeon, Percivall Pott, recognized the occupational hazard of scrotum cancer for young chimney sweeps. These unfortunate children, some as young as 4 years old, frequently crawled naked through chimneys both because of the heat and because nudity offered more flexibility. Pott's observation led to early legislation on health and occupation. A British parliamentary decree established a minimum age of 8 and specified a mandatory weekly bath to lessen the concentration of carcinogenic soot. As current discussion of tobacco use illustrates, the role of regulation of risk is still debated. Even later there would be consideration of psychosocial factors that may make individuals prone to cancer. In the comparatively prescientific pandemic of syphilis, venereal transmission was identified. Medical or psychological reasons might replace or supplement theological ones. But the end result was the same: The victims were responsible for their disease.

But these distinctions were not always so clear. Most diseases, even dreaded ones, evoked varied responses and drew on different images. For example, even tuberculosis had conflicting images. There were the romantic images of the lady of the "White Camellias" and the later movie "Camille" that evoked considerable sympathy for persons with tuberculosis. In such plays and literature, tuberculosis was a consumptive disease, striking at the beautiful and creative, evoking a powerful flowering even in the throes of death. That image, popular in literature, contrasted with other images of tuberculosis as a disease marked by consumption, sputum, and poverty. So as comforting and protective as this perspective of blaming the victim is, it clearly had exceptions; in some cases, the biography of a victim could easily allow the imputation of blame, whereas in other cases the life of the victim seemed exemplary. Children, even babies, suffered too from syphilis. Clearly, the disease afflicted both those deemed guilty and the innocent.

This led to a curious distinction between the deserving and undeserving. The vocabulary and language of the disease reflected that as well. As with AIDS, there were those that were considered "innocent" victims of disease. Sometimes spoken, other times unspoken, was the implied understanding that if some victims were identified as "innocent," others could be considered guilty.

This distinction is evident in leprosy. In the Old Testament, Leviticus does not judge the leper but does describe leprosy as unclean. But other passages (II Chronicles 26:16–23; Kings 15:1–6) do associate leprosy with some sin. Although some commentators debate whether these early references are, in fact, leprosy, medieval theologians, both Jewish and Christian, applied them to those currently diagnosed with leprosy. As Brody (1974) indicated, the medieval morality tales often related how someone chastised for sin by leprosy later repented and was cured. Leprosy was the result of alienation from God. Those who repented were restored.

Medieval commentators often described moral symptoms with the physical ones of leprosy. Lepers were angry, suspicious, scheming, and full of bad habits. Some commentators even identified the disease as sexually transmitted. An underlying theme was that lepers were lecherous, seeking to infect others through the close contact of sexual intercourse (Brody, 1974), a claim often advanced against persons with AIDS. These conceptions of the disease justified the harsh way victims of leprosy were treated. Stigmatized by a service reminiscent of a funeral, they were cast out of the community, restricted from major highways, and forced to warn all that approached.

This concept of leprosy was challenged by the Crusades. When some Crusaders returned from the Crusades afflicted with leprosy, another interpretation emerged. Some with leprosy were blessed with special grace, commending them to others so that others may show a blessed mercy. Again, morality tales reflected this. In one story, a monk carries a leper to a monastery, but the abbot who sees this act of charity miraculously sees the monk carrying Christ. Thus two attitudes are evident—the leper is sinner or saint. Even though the first attitude is more prevalent, a distinction is now evident between those deserving and those undeserving of the disease.

Syphilis, transmitted both natally and sexually, easily lent itself to such characterizations. The end of the 15th century, the time of the syphilis pandemic, was a sexually permissive era. Initially syphilis was seen by some as a mark of pride, a sign of masculinity. But as the horror of the disease unfolded and religious reformers railed against sexual license, it became more a mark of shame and sin than of sensuality. This too was reflected in fiction. A hit in the 1913 Broadway season, for example, was Brieux's *Damaged Goods*, a morality play of a young man who refuses to reveal his syphilis to his new wife. Both the wife and their child are later infected.

In that reformed time, as with HIV infection, both popular morality and literature build upon a distinction between those deserving of the disease and those undeserving innocent victims. When Thomas Parrin, the U.S. surgeon general, embraced a campaign against syphilis in 1936, his speeches tried to build public sympathy for victims by emphasizing clearly innocent, unsuspecting victims infected by *casual* transmission (Fee, 1988). It is interesting to see the gradual evolution of innocence. In the early years it is the innocent women, wives and virgins, who are inflicted with a terrible disease through the adulterous behavior of their husbands or the libertine irresponsibility of their betrothed. Later, especially in the 20th century, another link becomes added to this chain. In U.S. Army syphilis propaganda, it is unchaste women, particularly foreign prostitutes and promiscuous women, who are infecting thoughtless but essentially normal American males, who will then inadvertently infect their chaste women back home. These males then had to be protected by closing brothels, arresting and incarcerating prostitutes, and strengthening the laws against prostitution. As these distinctions between those deserving and undeserving sharpened, they were often reflected in policy. For example, during the last two World Wars, infected soldiers were treated punitively. This only encouraged silence, secrecy, and concealment, a protectiveness that impaired the Army's effectiveness in fighting infection.

Once one accepts the idea that there are those who deserve to be afflicted by the disease it becomes natural to label groups as well as individuals as deserving. After all, if certain individuals behave in ways that make them deserving of disease, so do groups of individuals share these negative attributes. Second, these judgments were supported by the observation that these different groups suffered disproportionately from the disease. Therefore, it could be reasoned that something lacking in their collective moral behavior or character was responsible. This too then served a defensive role, offering a psychological sense of protection that members of other groups would not suffer so, or if they did, that these other groups were to blame. Finally, such ideas could justify harsh actions against these groups. Here too these actions could be rationalized as simple measures of public health. The most obvious distinctions were those of class and ethnicity.

It did not take long to recognize that tuberculosis was more likely to afflict those in the lower classes. Although many reformers attributed this to social and economic conditions, others saw it as a reflection of a detestable lifestyle marked by alcoholism and a lack of hygiene. Even some of the reformist literature validated these ideas, claiming that effective change could not only raise social and economic conditions, but reform the poor habits of a depressed and oppressed lower class, improving their health, but also protecting the health of society at large. Living in the slums the poor could only maintain their dissolute habits, and remain living, breeding reservoirs of disease ready to affect society at large.

Because lower classes often suffered disproportionately from these diseases, many ethnic and racial groups, trapped in lower social classes, also suffered disproportionately. This, too, made them targets for blame. Already outcast, for these groups the disease became further evidence of inherent weakness and inferiority, either in constitution, habits, or morals.

Blaming other groups for disease has been a historically common response. Most of the epidemic plagues described in the previous chapter had been blamed on some malevolent act of an external enemy or internal suspect groups. "They," however they were defined, were responsible for causing or spreading the disease. Even syphilis was blamed on and named for a variety of external enemies. Here the group that suffered from the disease was now held responsible for it.

Syphilis and leprosy again provide illustration. Leprosy seems to have first appeared in the United States in New Orleans. Dr. A. Jones, the president of the Commission State Board of Health, blamed the Chinese, or in his words, "the filthy, vicious, debased, leprous Chinese," for this disease (Gussow, 1989, p. 56). To Jones, the practice of spitting out water by Chinese launderers in ironing was both detestable and unhealthy. Jones warned his countrymen that "patriots should contemplate with dread the overflow of their country by the unprincipled, vicious, leprous herders of Asia" (Gussow, 1989, p. 46).[5] Jones' concerns were echoed by others. The fear of leprosy was used as an argument against annexing Hawaii. Lurid speeches and articles questioned, "Should we annex leprosy?" Again the Chinese were blamed. The debates on immigration, particularly of Asians, were full of references to disease. In one, Oregon's Senator Salter charged that "the Chinese bring with them their filth, nameless diseases, and contagion" (Gussow, 1989, pp. 123–124). In California, where sinophobia was always an excellent vote pleaser, politicians claimed that the disease could even be spread by cigars wrapped by Chinese workers. Missionary literature, generally sympathetic to Asians, supported the stereotype. Donors were asked to give, not only to convert Chinese souls, but to save their bodies from loathsome diseases such as leprosy. The fact that non-Westerners, especially Asians, were identified with leprosy was further proof of Western superiority. In California and the West, where anti-Asian prejudice was high, the Chinese were also accused of sexual promiscuity and prostitution that certainly contributed to the spread of syphilis.

But in most other parts of the country, African Americans were castigated as a promiscuous race, hell-bent on spreading that disease. One book, written by Robert Shufeldt, a prominent southern surgeon and major in the Army Medical Corps, illustrates that theme. His highly racist 1915 book entitled *America's Greatest*

---

[5]Ironically, Jones's patriotism was never called into question, although he had been a Confederate officer during the Civil War.

Problem: The Negro characterized African Americans as a dying race spreading diseases such as syphilis and tuberculosis throughout the populace (McBride, 1991). The fact that many physicians characterized Blacks as—in the words of one—a "notoriously syphilis soaked" race (Jones, 1981) was perhaps one of the reasons the many Tuskegee syphilis experiments received little comment. In this study the U.S. Public Health Service deliberately withheld medical treatment for syphilis from 400 poor and illiterate African American males for 40 years (1932–1972) to see the ways that syphilis naturally unfolds. The men were merely told they had bad blood. They cooperated because they received free physicals, treatment for other minor ailments, and other small benefits. Because the study was poorly designed, little was learned from it. But it was no secret. Results, tracing the progressive illness of these men, were periodically reported in medical journals. This identification of race, sexuality, and syphilis was also used to argue for the continued segregation of Black soldiers. The legacy of this racist medicine still haunts in many ways the trust that African American groups and other minorities have in medical responses to HIV infection.

Blame was sometimes more subtle. Even when social behaviors or memberships in certain societal groups were not identified as worthy of blame, psychological attributes were. Recent work on cancer is an example of that. Although connections between social, psychological, and lifestyle factors and disease are valuable areas to be explored, one has to be careful of imputing blame on the victim. This is clear in lung cancer. Since the 1920s smoking has been identified as a factor in lung cancer. But as Patterson (1987) noted, only as more of the middle class gave up smoking did prohibitions on smoking gain ground. The identification of lifestyle factors or behaviors with disease again sharpens a societal distinction between those who deserve and those who do not deserve the disease. Already much of the language of the antismoking lobby supports such distinctions. They argue that you may choose to kill yourself (and thus deserve to die), but you have no right to poison the health of others (the nonsmokers affected by second-hand smoke). Perhaps in the future, the language of cancer will distinguish between innocent and, at least implied, deserving victims of disease. Again, because smoking behaviors differ among social classes and groups, class and ethnicity may become intertwined as well.

More recent and exciting work in cancer research and treatment focuses on psychological factors, such as personality types and their ability to handle stress, as causative factors in cancer. The attitudes and behaviors of patients in treatment are looked at as factors influencing their survival and this may also become a double-edged sword. On one hand this perspective may enable persons to take preventive actions to avert disease, and should they have the disease to become active participants in treatment. On the other hand, it can stigmatize persons with the disease as being psychologically weak, evidenced by both their illness and failure to respond.

Only polio has seemingly been exempt from stigma and blame. This disease attacked mainly children, and mostly middle class children were the ones that suffered. This turned the focus to the disease rather than the victim.

TREATING DISEASE

Given the sense of stigma and shame that these diseases evoke, it is unsurprising that persons with the disease were often segregated or compelled to suffer in silence. Again leprosy serves as an example. Once a person was suspected of having the disease, he or she was examined by an authority—at different times a priest or physician. If determined to have the disease, he or she was branded as a leper and separated from society—in leprosariums, lazar houses, or lazarettos. These extreme measures may have had some effectiveness. Richards (1977) credits this isolation as having had a significant role in eliminating the threat of leprosy in medieval Europe. But Richards (1977) too acknowledges that the bubonic plague may even have had a more effective role in eliminating leprosy from Western Europe. Even in the 19th and 20th centuries, this segregation continued. In the United States persons with leprosy were confined to a public hospital in Carville, Louisiana, or a leper colony in Molokai, Hawaii, creating their own distinct subculture. Yet the personal costs are hard to calculate. A recent anecdote, however, highlights these personal costs. Betty Martin, now 87, once a New Orleans debutante, was diagnosed with leprosy. After changing her name, her family shipped her off to Carville, leaving her disappearance a local mystery. Isolated in the walls she recounts that even there the sense of stigma never left. She tells the story of listening to the 1937 World Series on the radio. After a bad call, the announcer called the umpire "the leper" of the game, saying "Nobody touches him, everyone despises him."

The segregation that persons with leprosy suffered varied from culture to culture and time to time. For example, although varied regulations restricted lepers in India, the culturally similar and geographically near island of Sri Lanka did not so segregate victims of leprosy. Sometimes, too, political events affected treatment. Newly independent Norway, faced with a persistent problem with leprosy among their poor, mandated isolation of lepers in the Act of 1885. Yet this segregation was never rigorously enforced nor were victims stigmatized. Lepers were perceived sympathetically as impoverished and neglected Norwegians. In this time of nascent nationalism, the model of care sought to be humane and rational.

Victims of other stigmatic diseases also faced extensive segregation and discrimination. At times many hospitals refused to treat syphilis, polio, or tuberculosis patients. Again, although the conditions for the rich were tolerable, the poor's accommodations were much worse. Saranac Lake, in New York's Adirondack Mountains, which housed a sanatorium for the well-to-do, was avoided as a "city of the sick," but Raybrook, a sanatorium for indigent persons in nearby Lake Placid, was perceived as a virtual leper colony. Both had problems attracting medical help. In both towns, patients visiting the town might be greeted by signs reading "No Tuberculars," forbidding them to enter stores. Polio and cancer victims were also isolated in special hospitals and wards, and in these cases their previous residence was often stripped and their possessions were discarded and burned.

Given the fear and reaction these diseases engendered, victims often chose to suffer in silence. In some cases the silence was necessary and protective. For example, because U.S. soldiers were treated punitively for contracting syphilis, many chose to hide symptoms or seek treatment privately. This silence even extended, in some diseases, past death itself. Many who died from cancer were listed in obituaries as having died from a "long illness"; the dreaded word "cancer" was simply too awful to say. Perhaps, as mentioned earlier, the major reason that use of that euphemistic phrase has declined is simply families fear it may be misinterpreted now as AIDS.

Class and gender sometimes mediated responses to disease. Upper class persons, especially men, could escape on clipper ships or to the frontier to seek more compatible climes. Upper class women could at least seek the "resting cure" in tolerable sanitoriums. It was the poor who were confined to less than desirable hospitals or died abandoned in their homes.

This silence complicated treatment. In many ways conflicts over the treatment of these diseases finds echoes in AIDS. These diseases were so stigmatizing that infected persons and their families desired secrecy. Yet public health needs often compromised that desire for secrecy, setting up a series of conflicts between individual and collective rights.

One of the earliest conflicts was over the need to report the disease. In a very real sense, leprosy was the first reportable disease. Those with knowledge of a suspected leper were expected to report that fact to authorities so the suspected victim could be examined. Much later, many U.S. states required physicians to report either tuberculosis or syphilis, raising conflicts for physicians over respective responsibilities to individual patients or a perceived public good. Beyond the threat to privacy, reportability of disease raised a host of other issues still evident in HIV infection. How well could the confidentiality of the report be maintained? What actions could result from the report? If the consequences of the report were so dire, would those suspecting evidence of disease be reluctant to seek medical help—thus not only complicating their own treatment but possibly endangering the health of others?

The disease also raised other rights issues. Does a government have the right to restrict the rights of an individual with the disease to protect the health of others? In the medieval era, questions were rarely if at all raised. The concept of individual rights was limited and restricted. But as the concept of individual rights grew, questions began to be raised: What powers did agencies and governments possess? How well could they enforce quarantines or other restrictive measures? Could they compel inoculations or restricted access to schools because children were not inoculated? For example, in one of the early epidemics of polio, New York City Health Commissioner Dr. Emerson stated, "The early control, not only of poliomyelitis, but of all preventable diseases, does not depend on the mysterious powers of any supernatural agency, but lies largely within ourselves" (Paul, 1971, p. 157). Emerson, like many public health figures of the time, favored vigorous actions to enforce public health measures, even going so far as to remove a child from parental care when the parents seemed unable or unwilling to maintain quarantine.

As stated earlier, there was a constant tension between those who saw such actions as regrettable but necessary responses to crisis and those who disagreed. For example, British attempts to mandate smallpox inoculation in 1853 and 1867 aroused stiff opposition. In fact, in 1867 an antivaccination league formed to campaign against mandatory inoculation. Its members raised various arguments— inoculation was unproven or dangerous, it interfered with the rights of parents, it was a violation of liberty, it was unworkable because many disregarded the law. Subsequent laws in 1898 and 1907 allowed parents the right to conscientously object (Porter & Porter, 1988). Yet in many ways these disagreements were not merely a philosophical expression of the primacy of individual rights over collective good. Often they were based on the practical assumption that such actions were counterproductive.

Nowhere was this more evident than in the debates over the treatment of syphilis. Syphilis was intertwined not only with issues of health and prevention but with morality and sexuality. From the beginning, then, there were conflicts between moralistic and pragmatic approaches. As early as 1500 Spanish physicians were suggesting that prostitutes be inspected and regulated, while religious reformers were using syphilis as an argument that prostitutes should be rigorously suppressed. Even in the 20th century, there were conflicts over providing condoms and sex education to soldiers or attempting to rigorously enforce appropriate moral conduct. In these more secular times, syphilis pitted two modern concepts against one another—a Freudian concept of the id that saw the sex drive as difficult to control, versus a progressive belief in the individual's ability to change and direct behavior. Some moralists even bemoaned penicillin as a last blow to morality.

The fact that syphilis could be transmitted through intimate social contact or congenitally raised other issues. Should sexual partners be informed? Should blood tests be required for marriage or for expectant mothers? Underlying these debates was a question with profound moral implications: What role did the state have in protecting those deemed blameless—innocent spouses and children—from the sins of those perceived as guilty? These conflicts, never fully resolved, continue to haunt policy on AIDS.

CONCLUSION

In many ways, this review of stigmatic disease affirms both the possibilities and limits of science. The responses to many of these diseases represent triumphs of medicine. Smallpox seems eradicated. Polio and leprosy, dreaded diseases of times past, seem in the West remote memories. Tuberculosis, until its reemergence with AIDS, was, at least in the West, on the wane. Syphilis is no longer a cause of great concern, only an occasion for a shot of penicillin. Even cancer, still a major killer, has lost some of its fearful opprobrium.

Yet these diseases all show the limits of science as well. The history of each disease offers a reminder of the ways that fear powerfully influences both medical treatment and public health policy. And they are a reminder that at times these fears inhibit both humane and effective responses to disease.

Chapter **3**

LESSONS UNLEARNED: THE DREADED DISEASES IN HISTORY

People and government have never learned anything from history or acted on principles derived from it.
                                    Hegel, Philosophy of History

If there is one lesson we can learn from the history of dreaded diseases, it is the truth of Hegel's insight. With an almost hopeless, inevitable repetitiveness, the same themes are constantly reenacted. A disease emerges to be defined as "dread." That fear and repulsion institute a predictable cycle of events that both isolate those who suffer from the disease and impose an effective, societal response. The irrational fear drives policy. The loathing determines treatment.

In a sense, the critical question is "What can be learned from the history of dreaded diseases that might shape an effective response to this new epidemic?" As the succeeding chapters indicate, the answer might very well be, at least up to now, "not much." Patterns of denial and avoidance were and remain prevalent responses to AIDS. As in the past, there is an ongoing hope, which almost seems to drive policy, that suggests that AIDS will always remain a disease of the marginalized groups or sections of the world that it now affects. As before, AIDS has challenged any conception of community, exposing fault lines in societies as each group blames others for the disease or response. There is no consensus on ways to maintain the balance between collective and individual rights. And as long as persons with the disease suffer the stigma of a dreaded disease, effective public health responses will be limited.

This chapter explores that dreadful cycle. It begins by developing the concept of a dreaded disease, examining the ways that fear and loathing are reflected and perpetuated in image and metaphor. Second, it considers the definitional cycle of a disease. What factors cause a disease to be labeled as especially abhorrent? What factors cause such irrational fear to abate? Third, the chapter reviews the implications of dreaded diseases—the ways and direction blame is cast and the implications of fear for the development of policy.

THE CONCEPT OF A DREADED DISEASE

During the heart of the desegregation struggles, Dick Gregory, an African American satirist, used to recount a telling anecdote. It seems a major segregationist, whoever was in the forefront of hate at the moment, had visited his physician. The doctor somberly told him he had bad news and worse news. "Give me the bad news first," the segregationist asks. The physician replies, "You've got a terminal disease that will slowly kill you." "Oh, my God," the man responds, "What can be worse than that?" "It's sickle cell anemia," Gregory deadpans.

The anecdote reemphasizes a point made throughout the preceding chapters —that each disease has a meaning. Whereas sickle cell anemia and similar conditions may define one's ethnicity, other diseases may define one's character or sin. There is an interactive quality to these definitions. The ways a disease defines its victims affect the ways the disease itself is defined. Diseases that carry an opprobrium are readily dreaded.

But sometimes the opprobrium is collective. The judgments of the great epidemic diseases, the plagues, were not so much on an individual. The death toll was too massive to allow that interpretation, and far too seemingly random. They were a judgment on the larger society. It was the society as a whole that needed to be chastised—though even during the plagues there were groups of sinners that could be blamed for calling down judgment.

The fact that these diseases were defined differently, in frightening terms, is reflected in the languages and metaphors. Susan Sontag (1978, 1988), in her works on illness and metaphor, indicated the ways that language and meaning of disease constantly affected one another. Certain diseases take on metaphoric meanings because they are so dreaded in a particular time and culture. We speak of an outcast as a "leper," a curse as a "pox." Cancer becomes a metaphor for any slow, uncontrollable, invasive force, whether it's perceived as poverty or communism, that saps at the health of its host society. Any horrendous event we define as a plague. Syphilis conveys a sense of denigration of the soul.

Sometimes the name of the disease itself is metaphoric. Although the "Black Death" refers to some of the physical symptomatology of the disease, it simultaneously refers to something deeper and darker. The color black often has been associated with darkness and evil. To die of the Black Death conveys a sense of disturbing judgment. "Cancer" also is a metaphoric name. Drawn from the name of the crab, it is unclear whether the ancients alluded to its slow tenacity, the painfulness of its bite, or the shape of common tumors.

Whereas the metaphors reflect the fear the disease conveyed, they also reflect back upon the victim. To have a disease with that name conveys all the meanings of the name itself. The disease becomes a key social identity, often submerging other aspects of the self. Preston (1979) told of the "Gregor Effect." Using the name of the character Gregor from Kafka's *Metamorphosis*, he develops an analogy with that story. Gregor awoke one morning to find he was trapped in the body of a roach. But it's his family's treatment of him as a loathsome insect that completes the transition. Only when he is treated as less than human does Gregor truly become an insect in self as well as appearance. To Preston, a disease can have the same effect. Being a cancer victim can overwhelm all other identities. It is the disease by which one is identified.

When the person has a dreaded disease this Gregor effect can be devastating. All the meanings that the disease conveys are now translated to the person. The person is now considered a victim, a leper, a syphilitic.

The name of the disease can be so steeped in meaning that ultimately it becomes an impediment to treatment. Leprosy had so many, almost primal, connotations of dread and loathsomeness that advocates for the disease, both those who suffered it and others, sought to change the name. They believed the treatment of leprosy could never be medicalized, and the treatment of those with the disease humanized, as long as the disease's name remained.

Sometimes the meanings can be ambivalent, even exotic. Tuberculosis was the dreaded "White Death." Here even the name hinted at ambivalence. There was another side to tuberculosis, an image of romanticism, images of a young girl, a Camille, wasting away, beautiful in her consumption, or of a poet whose creative juices are fed by impending death. The image contrasted with the other more pervasive image—a disease of the slums, brought on, depending on one's ideology, by overwork or alcoholism, one more horror of the inner cities. Syphilis provides another example. As stated earlier, syphilis too had ambivalent meanings. In its early times it was a badge of manhood until the full long-term effects of the disease became clear. And once an easy cure was found, the dread receded and the earlier ambivalent meaning of the disease returned. Yet the gender differential is amplified as well. Although there were times that syphilis was a badge of manhood, it never was a mark of womanhood. The woman with syphilis was either pitied as an innocent despoiled by an unfaithful lover or despised as a whore.

THE DEFINITION OF A DISEASE AS DREAD

This process of defining the disease is not random. It is rooted in the nature of the disease, the efficacy of treatment, and in the time itself. Aires (1987) recounted that human orientations toward death change. In medieval times, it was the sudden death that was feared. Such a death gave no time to prepare for death, to make peace with God in a time so judgmental in its theology. The lack of suffering offered no recompense for the torments of purgatory. In such a society the Black Death, with its rapid descent into death, would generate intense fear.

Other diseases generated dread, in part because they were beyond history. By this it is meant that the affected society believed that such diseases could no longer strike them. In a sense the disease forced the afflicted societies to re-evaluate their position in the world. Both the influenza pandemic of 1918–1919 and the cholera epidemic challenged Western and American society's assumptive sense of reality. In the mid-18th century, the Western world, the United States in particular, looked at the cholera epidemic, beginning in India, as a sign of the primitive. Their own advanced societies they perceived as immune. The disease toppled that arrogance, reaffirming in its horror a common biology and humanity. Similarly, the influenza epidemic devastated a society that believed that the age of epidemics was now over and science could control such a minor thing as the flu. The HIV epidemic too is partially dreaded for that very reason. Many believed that Western society could not fall prey to a viral infectious epidemic.

Demographics of disease too can add to the sense of dread. Some diseases were feared because they were so random. But others were dreaded because they struck so atypically. Both syphilis and influenza, much like HIV, felled young adults, who were perceived as reasonably safe from diseases, having survived childhood illness and still immune to the ravages of age. McNeill (1976) reminded us that epidemics that kill young adults often have a significant impact on society. Because such epidemics affect those who are most productive, they can cause severe economic dislocation. But even more important, such diseases seem to demoralize and spiritually deplete these societies.

It is unsurprising that there is a cultural component to dread as well. Each culture can define dread differently. The differences in culture, however small, are distinct enough that the same disease is defined differently.

There is also a social component to disease. Some diseases were dreaded because they threatened the social order. The disease brought in its wake massive mortality, and chaos or at least the threat of chaos. Other diseases were dreaded because they identified an individual with more marginal social groups. Either the disease made one an outcast (such as leprosy) or affirmed that one was an outcast (such as syphilis).

However the cultural, social, historical, or demographic context frames the definition of the disease, characteristics of the disease are critical in defining a disease as dread. As stated in earlier chapters, dreaded diseases are of two types. The feared contagious diseases were generally fatal, quick and unpredictable, contagious, and the cause of considerable mortality, decimating communities. The stigmatic diseases were disfiguring, slow, painful, debilitating, progressively chronic, and externally manifest.

In addition, uncertainty as to how a disease is transmitted also contributes to a sense of dread. When the mode of transmission is uncertain, either because medical science has not yet developed theories of transmission or because the disease occurred at a time in history when medicine was very limited, every act and each person is a potential source of danger. However, transmission can be uncertain even when science is sure. There are two reasons for this seeming paradox. First, throughout history there have been times when the medical profession has been distrusted, particularly by certain segments of society. Often it has been those segments, especially the poor and marginalized groups, that have been most ravaged by disease. If medical science is not to be trusted, physicians' theories of transmission will make little difference to a disbelieving population. In the early years of AIDS, a joking interpretation of the acronym AIDS was "An Imaginary Disease Discouraging Sex." This distrust of the medical establishment is evident in cancer as well, as witnessed by the cancer counterculture. It will later be seen as a contributory factor to the panic generated by AIDS.

Second, the language of science is by its very nature not a language of certainty. Rather it is a language of probabilities. To a population desperate for certain reassurance, affirmations of remote probability are likely to be received as ambiguous and offer little comfort. The assertion that there is little chance, a statement as clear as the language of probability allows, may be interpreted as "no chance" by someone familiar with the uncertainty of scientific language. But to a person unfamiliar with those nuances, it opens possibilities one would rather be closed.

Two other factors of a disease add a sense of dread. First is the onset. Most dreaded diseases had an insidious onset. The initial symptoms could signify any range of illnesses. Nonspecific as the symptoms were, they increased a sense of uncertainty and anxiety. Second, a treatment too was uncertain. In some diseases little could be done at all. But when something could be done, it was often tedious, painful, and uncertain as to whether it could control or cure the disease. When treatment or prevention became perceived as effective, the sense of dread often abated.

This discussion reaffirms a major point. The dread of a disease is rooted in a historical and social context. Meanings of disease are open to change as conditions change. Dread is specific to place, time, and context.

Once a disease is dreaded, there is only a small step to irrational, panicked reactions. The fact that a disease is feared is a precondition for panic. Fear of a disease alone is not sufficient to create panic, but it does create the necessary conditions for panic to occur if other factors are present.

Smelser (1963) in his "value-added" theory of collective behavior noted three factors necessary for panic. Panic is only possible when all three conditions are fulfilled. The first is a "structural conduciveness." This is a society that is often in a state of flux, transition. In this context there is a general feeling of unease and ambiguity. Most of the panicked reactions that greeted the dreaded diseases took place when the social structure was itself in transition. For example, the bubonic plague struck when the established orders of the time, the Roman empire of feudal order, were themselves undergoing transition. Cholera emerged at the time of the industrial revolution. Other epidemics, like influenza, emerged at a time of war. In these times there is often a deep-seated sense of anxiety, an uneasiness, a feeling of threat. And in these times there is often a distrust of authority. Their information and responses are distrusted.

A second condition is a "precipitating incident," something that seems to confirm the threat or give face to the underlying anxiety. In some cases it is evidence that the new disease has reached or struck close to home. For example, it may be that there is a report that cases of the disease have begun to emerge in one's own city or neighborhood. It may be a rumor that the disease is spread by a particular product or person. In any case, an event occurs that allows individuals to focus their fears.

Finally, there is a mobilization for flight. Here there is a departure from established behavior that provides supportive permission for other panicked behaviors. For example, one person neglecting his or her role or fleeing provides support for each other person selecting to do so.

Widespread panics tended to be more characteristic of the epidemic plagues. In the stigmatic diseases responses were more local. Panics would occur but these tended to be restricted in area. However, often a disease would have a defining moment, a time when it seemed to reach public notice, a moment where the private suffering emerged as a general threat evoking fear. Cancer provides an apt illustration. Cancer was a long-standing disease dating back to antiquity. Yet the fear of cancer emerged as a powerful threat in the late 19th century. It was a conducive time. Cancer seemed a metaphor for the era—an uncontrollable, invasive growth that seemed relentless and impersonal. But it was U.S. President Ulysses Grant's death that brought cancer from a private affair to a social issue. AIDS, too, comes at a conducive time. The concept of systems breaking down, prey to whatever exists on the outside, the result of a hidden, unseen infection, strikes a sensitive chord in many societies at the end of the 20th century, one that now merits public concern and societal action.

THE IMPLICATIONS OF A DREADED DISEASE

Once a disease is dreaded, there is often a search to blame some group. In many cases the blame is externalized. Some groups, whether foreign or domestic enemies, are blamed. In some cases, these opponents are seen as deliberately spreading the disease. In other cases, others are seen as responsible for the disease, even if they are not perceived as consciously seeking to spread the disease. For example, an accusation was implied in the Spanish flu or the "French disease" (for syphilis). Here the assumption was that the spread of disease was not deliberate, but nonetheless, another society was to blame for their dissolute habits or backwardness. These societies not only brought the disease on themselves, but on other, more worthy societies as well. This pattern is very clear in AIDS. The toll of the disease, its entry in socially marginal groups, the modern common belief that new diseases and epidemics are a past relic, and research in genetic engineering convinced many that this disease was not a natural occurrence, but an intentional or unintentional effect of science. On occasion, some blame may be accepted by the collectivity as a whole. In that case, the disease is defined as a chastisement.

It is a small step to blame the victim. This blame could be for spreading the disease, often malevolently. The assumption was that those who had the disease conspired to bring others into misery. Blame, too, was placed on victims for their condition. Claiming that those who had the disease deserved it served two functions. First, it gave meaning to the event. An incomprehensible horror became understandable. The disease could be interpreted within the social context. Second, it was protective. The thought that only those who deserved the disease received it alleviated anxiety. If one lived right or prayed right, one was protected from illness.

With AIDS, blame was especially easy to apportion. After all, the affected groups—IV drug users, homosexuals, and prostitutes—were all groups that generally were perceived within parts of society to have low social standing. Prostitutes are a particularly interesting case. Prostitutes clearly seem to be a vector of disease in certain circumstances. Prostitutes who are IV drug users have high rates of infection. In Africa, where condoms tend not to be used for economic and cultural reasons, prostitutes certainly play a significant role in the spread of the disease. In the West, however, beyond these poor streetwalkers, prostitutes do not seem to have high rates of seropositivity, or play a significant role in spreading HIV (Richardson, 1988). Again, as in the case of syphilis, the blame on prostitutes and calls for restrictiveness reinforce the image of the unclean woman spreading disease. As syphilis led to acts against prostitutes and the closing of brothels, a curious double standard is evident. The role of the male customer is ignored.

Once blame was apportioned, punitive policies could be implemented. In some cases these served to expel or isolate those suspected of spreading the disease, wittingly or unwittingly. These policies may be neither rational nor necessarily effective. Responding more to political, social, and moral definitions than medical realities, they did little good and sometimes great harm.

Yet these policies emphasized a critical point. Medical policies are not shaped in a vacuum. A dreaded disease is a social, political, and moral event. It is a moral event insofar as those suffering from disease carry a moral definition. In rare cases, that definition may be positive as in the heroic cast of children suffering from polio or leper crusaders. But more often than not, the moral definition is negative. Victims of the disease are portrayed as weak, unworthy, and immoral. These moral definitions have a twofold effect. First, they inhibit early detection and treatment. Given the definitions of the disease, few wish to openly acknowledge their condition. Second, these moral definitions justify punitive treatments. This also becomes self-defeating. As punitive sanctions rise, there is even more incentive toward secrecy and deception.

Dreaded diseases are also political events where policies are developed in the political arena, which is again more shaped by fear, so more extreme and punitive measures are often favored.

This too complements the general social mood. Diseases that strike great fear demand extraordinary responses. The fear that the disease arouses powerfully shapes both public health policies and medical treatment. For example, the quarantines of bubonic plague victims were suggested more by fear than coherent medical theory. And sometimes quarantines were so total that even life-giving medications could not be sent.

There are also countervailing forces that seek to minimize the threat. First there are the forces of optimism and inertia. Humans often cope with potential threat by minimizing it, and, in essence, hoping it will recede on its own. There is always a force that seeks to believe even in the midst of disease that an epidemic has run its course or a disease is less of a threat than perceived. Therefore there is little need to change stable patterns of interaction or established norms. This is often buttressed by a second force, economic interests. Any drastic change in the social order will often be resisted by those economic powers invested in that order. Because any response to disease threatens the status quo, economic interests often seek to minimize any potential or actual threat. As one views the history of these diseases, the voice of these interests was often one of caution. Sometimes this caution was beneficial as it minimized irrational responses. Sometimes it was dysfunctional as it inhibited any responses to an emergent crisis.

In summation, as long as a disease is so deeply dreaded, responses to that disease, shaped more by political, social, and moral forces, are likely to be both nonrational and ineffective. Only when this fear abates—either because the threat recedes or the treatment becomes more effective—is the disease likely to be viewed as a medical issue, where treatment and policy are shaped more by public health concerns than other forces. This is not to imply that that ever fully happens. Any disease will be affected by moral, social, and political considerations. But in diseases that are socially "dreaded," it is that fear more than anything else that shapes a response.

CONCLUSION

There is much that can be learned from our past encounters with dreaded diseases that might be applied to AIDS. Specifically, if dreaded diseases from the past teach us anything, two lessons are critical. The first is that we need to understand and to break the cycle of fear that inhibits an effective response to the disease. Second, we have to recognize the disease, rather than one another, as the foe. Only such a recognition will allow a common response to this new public health threat.

There is one additional lesson that history teaches. The emergence of these dreaded diseases tended to take place at times when social conditions and processes were in transition. Wars, periods of significant trade, changes in transportation, or large movements of people became vectors for a disease to emerge. Other changes, too, in economic or social organization or in sexual or social mores were often factors in the emergence and spread of disease. There is a neglected sociology of disease that reminds us that when the conditions of social life change it disturbs the fragile equilibrium that exists between humans and the microorganisms with which we coexist. This equilibrium is always in dynamic tension. When humans first walked upright into the savannas, perhaps even to flee the disease of the tropics, this balance was challenged. Every innovation in technology—from the domestication of animals to the cultivation of grain— upsets that tentative relationship, bringing in its wake new diseases. Patterns of trade change, new modes of interaction and interrelationships merge, old diseases are conquered—and all of these events create or expand niches for microbes, some perhaps evolving themselves. This fragile dance between species is likely to continue until the end of time, whether the time of humans or, perhaps even more unlikely, the time of these microbes. Although humankind often ignores that tentative relationship it has with the ever larger unseen environment, we disturb it at our peril.

PART II
AIDS:
THE ARCHETYPE
OF THE DREADED DISEASES

Chapter 4

THE NATURE AND ORIGIN
OF AIDS

*We had no such thing as printed newspapers in those days to
spread rumors and reports of things, and to improve them by
the invention of men, as I have lived to see practiced since.*
Defoe, Journal of the Plague Years

In the late 1900s, a new disease, at least newly perceived, emerged into the
consciousness of the world. Within a decade, that disease would be as dreaded
as any disease in the past. Whereas the first victims of the previous dreaded
diseases remain anonymous, the names and histories of the first persons with
AIDS in the United States are known. Yet this belies the fact that AIDS' first
victims were also unrecognized and as anonymous as any of the victims of earlier
diseases and plagues. The origins and onset of AIDS are currently disputed. But
as the disease unfolded over time, it gradually became both recognized and feared.

This chapter chronicles the history of this disease. It begins by reviewing the
early days of its presence in the United States, noting both the initial recognition
of the disease and the initial responses the disease provoked. The chapter then
explores and evaluates the African hypothesis of the origin of AIDS. This hypothesis is interesting for two reasons. First, it has interesting echoes of previous
responses to dreaded diseases, that is, blaming others. Second, it obscures the
critical reasons for the emergence of AIDS. Whatever the origins of AIDS, it was
changing social conditions that allowed the disease to develop and to spread so
rapidly.

Finally, this chapter considers the reasons why the disease, once it was recognized, conjured such great fear and dread. It is the thesis of this section that AIDS is in many ways the archetype of the dreaded disease, a composite of all the factors that have in the past generated a sense of panic and dread. The implications of that dread will be the subject of subsequent chapters.

THE CRISIS UNFOLDS

The first official recognition of a new disease was obscure enough. On June 5, 1981, the Centers for Disease Control (CDC) noted it in its *Morbidity and Mortality Weekly Report* in a brief article entitled "Pneumocystis Carinii Pneumonia in Los Angeles." The article was a response to a CDC query about a comparative rash of requests for pentamidine, a drug used to treat *Pneumocystis carinii* pneumonia (PCP). Because the disease was so rare and generally the result of some immune suppression, the CDC's interest was tweaked by what was a significant increase in requests for pentamidine, especially because the cause of the immune suppression was unknown. More than that, some of these requests were for a second treatment with the drug. In typical use the drug worked initially and no further treatment was necessary. Although the report noted the disease among a population of young males, it only marginally referred to the fact that all these young men were gay. Shilts (1987) claimed that this reticence was caused by a desire to neither offend the gay community nor inflame homophobic sentiments both within and outside the medical establishment.

The CDC report officially recognized a problem that had slowly been observed over the previous 2 years. Physicians in New York, San Francisco, and Los Angeles had been noticing a series of strange medical conditions in their gay clientele, such as unexplained fevers, night sweats, diarrhea, and enlarged lymph nodes. More ominously, in 1979, a young, gay, New York school teacher, Rick Wellikoff, was diagnosed with a strange form of skin cancer, Kaposi's sarcoma (KS). This disease is traditionally found in Africa or among older Jewish and Italian men. Outside of Africa KS tended to be fairly benign and generally not life-threatening. Yet in this case, and in similar cases that began to appear, the disease seemed far more virulent. These men too showed signs of immune system suppression. There seemed only one common factor. All were promiscuous gay men. Ironically many of them knew each other or shared mutual friends. By July 4, 1981, the CDC's *Mortality and Morbidity Weekly Report* recognized 26 cases of KS, noting that some of these cases also exhibited PCP or other signs of immune deficiency. The CDC found the number of cases of KS disturbingly high and the association between the disease and sexual preference puzzling. By the end of 1981, CDC reports were even more troubling. The disease had been spreading from initial cities of Los Angeles, New York, and San Francisco. The appearance of this yet unnamed syndrome in intravenous (IV) drug users suggested a frightening possibility—this disease was caused by an infectious agent and, like hepatitis B, could be spread by blood products or through sexual contact.[1]

The response of both the government and the medical establishment to this unfolding crisis is likely to be long debated. That they were slow to respond is not debatable. Perrow and Guillen (1990) note that from the very beginning funding for research, care, and education was woefully inadequate. Congress earmarked more than President Ronald Reagan requested, and even later spent, to fight or prevent this new disease. Private foundations began to offer support in 1983, 2 years after the disease was identified. The blood industry denied any possibility of risk from blood supplies for almost half a year after the CDC raised suspicions that AIDS was blood-borne. And movements to close significant vectors of infection like the bathhouses would be fought more than 3 years after the disease was identified.

The reasons for this are far more complex than simple homophobia. Homophobia clearly was a factor. The fact that the disease seemed to strike marginalized and unpopular groups mitigated any general claim for research. Grmek (1990) describes some of the cruel humor that characterized such blatant homophobia. For example, one comedian noted that "the disease affects homosexual men, drug users, and Haitians. Thank God it hasn't spread to human beings yet." Another suggested that the disease be called WOGS—"Wrath of God Syndrome."

Possibly more destructive was the more subtle homophobia. Physicians and politicians knew little about gay lifestyle practices. In some cases, they may have been reluctant to become identified with a disease that was popularly defined as a gay or homosexual illness. For example, Shilts (1987) suggests that one of the reasons that New York City was slow to offer services or to even recognize the needs of its gay men with AIDS was that Mayor Edward Koch, a single male who had been the victim of a prior election whispering campaign claiming he was gay,

---

[1]Readers who wish a more comprehensive history of the disease may find two excellent books. Grmek (1990) offers a classic and scholarly account of the history of the disease. Shilts (1987) provides a more partisan but highly regarded and well-written journalistic diary of the AIDS crisis.

was averse to taking a leadership role on an issue so clearly defined as gay in the public mind.

But homophobia was only part of the reason for the delayed response. The AIDS epidemic struck in the opening years of the Reagan administration. The election of Ronald Reagan as president in 1980 represented no less than a major shift in the political paradigm. In contrast to prior administrations, a central thesis in the Reagan ideology was that the role of the federal government needed to be dramatically reduced. In this era of extensive budget cuts, gay political capital to increase funding for their own agenda was severely limited.

There were three reasons for this. First, the Republican coalition that elected Reagan included a component of the fundamentalist religious right. To this group, homosexuality was anathema. Some members of this faction were actively hostile to gays. For example, conservative columnist and later presidential candidate Pat Buchanan would write at the onset of the AIDS epidemic:

> The sexual revolution has begun to devour its children. And among the revolutionary vanguard, the gay rights activists, the morality rate is highest and climbing. . . . The poor homo-sexuals—they have declared war on nature and now nature is exacting an awful retribution. (quoted in Shilts, 1983, p. 311)

This opinion was not shared by all in the religious right; many were silent, some even compassionate. But, there was an antipathy to accepting anything that was perceived as a gay agenda. A basic political point of the moralistic and religious right was that the government could not condone homosexual behavior. Acknowledging the gay lobby was tantamount to embracing homosexuality.

There was a second political factor as well. Although American gay men, like other Americans, spanned the political spectrum, gay political activists and the gay establishment were publicly identified as members of the Democratic Party coalition. At the time, all of the congressmen openly identified as gay were Democrats. Hence the gay political establishment had little entry and even less clout with a conservative Republican administration. Other groups such as IV drug users were even more marginalized and powerless.

Finally, the gay community was itself fragmented. In the initial years of the epidemic, some gays believed that talk of a "gay cancer" or other gay-related disease was simply an expression of homophobic physicians that should be resisted lest gay sex be perceived as unhealthy. On a larger level the gay community's primary political focus had been to minimize the government's role in their life—for example, repealing sodomy laws, ending practices that discriminated against homosexuals, and permitting the functioning of gay establishments such as bars and bathhouses. It was now difficult to get a consensus that the government needed to take a more activist role. This lack of consensus was echoed in many minority communities, also struck by AIDS, and equally reluctant to acknowledge an emerging problem.

Even if the monies had been made available, the medical establishment may have been unable to effectively absorb it. Despite the outbreak of a series of viral diseases such as Ebola, Lassa, and Marburg fevers, the attention of the medical establishment had turned from acute disease to the management of chronic disease. Much like the hubris, a false pride, that preceded cholera, there was a perception that viral plagues were an artifact of the past. Communicable disease now had low research priority.

Then, too, there is an inherent conservatism in scientific research. Divisions of the National Institutes of Health had long established areas of responsibility with established research agents and protocols. Even under the best of circumstances, it would take 9 months to go through funding procedures. Medical researchers too had developed their own areas of expertise and lines of research. For these reasons, it would be difficult to change gears to accommodate a new disease. One clear lesson of the AIDS epidemic was that the medical establishment was generally unprepared and unsuited for a new medical emergency. This was something that Congress tried to rectify by setting up a $30 million reserve fund for public health emergencies (Panem, 1985).

The early theories about AIDS did not encourage researchers to begin work in the area. In the very beginning there was a suspicion, born of the intimate connections between the early victims, that this was a disease more readily solved by medical sleuths probing into lifestyle factors and/or an infectious source, than one demanding basic scientific research. The early theories of the disease varied. Because many in the early clusters of victims shared common environments such as bathhouses, some theorized that perhaps, much as in Legionnaires' Disease, something faulty in a bathhouse such as the ventilation system might be responsible for the appearance of this strange syndrome.

Others considered aspects of the sexual experience. Many of the early victims of the disease reported using "poppers" or amyl butyl nitrates, a drug frequently used as an inhalant to heighten sexual pleasure. Perhaps a batch had somehow gone bad. Others suggested that some aspect of the homosexual experience might be responsible. Because semen has immunosuppressive qualities, some hypothesized that the large amounts of semen in the body might break down the immune system. Others suggested an "immune overload" theory. Because the earliest victims were highly sexually active, many had experienced multiple bouts with varied infections and sexually transmitted diseases over the years. It was theorized that at some time the immune system simply broke down after multiple onslaughts with repeated invasion. Some even suggested that perhaps if there was a genetic trait for homosexuality that there might also be a different genetic configuration to the immune system (Altman, 1986).

Still other theories emphasized co-infections of common viruses. For example, Duesberg (1989) viewed AIDS as a combination of conventional viruses (such as Epstein-Barr and herpes) that operated in conjunction with lifestyle practices. These connections were explored by others as well. One of the first physicians working in the area thought that the early symptoms of AIDS, soon identified as AIDS-related complex (ARC), such as fever, swollen lymph nodes, and weight loss were manifestations of cytomegalovirus (CMV), a member of the herpes family and endemic in the gay community. All of these initial theories shared a common thread—that the cause of this new disease was likely to be found in the particular experiences of this cluster of early patients. Thus massive investments of time or research were not encouraged.

Legionnaires' Disease is often given as a reason for this initial lack of interest in what would soon be called AIDS. This disease first came to public attention in 1976, when there was an outbreak of pneumonia among American legionnaires attending a conference in Philadelphia. There were 182 stricken by disease and, of those, 29 died. Although the disease generated great attention at the CDC, two points must be considered. First, there was an ongoing concern that an antigen shift in the influenza virus might herald a new form of influenza similar to the form that caused 1918–1919 epidemic. This fear similarly fueled the panic to produce a swine flu vaccine at the same time. This outbreak of disease among 182 men who had little in common except a brief period of proximity generated fear that a new disease might have developed that was both highly infectious and often fatal. The shared histories and comparatively slow initial onslaught of AIDS did not generate that same panic. Second, the fact that the organism that caused the disease, *Legionella pneumophilia*, was found to be spread through the ventilation systems reinforced the notion that the cause of AIDS would likely be found to be similarly pedestrian, thus not encouraging medical researchers to alter their present research plans.

Although perhaps the delay is understandable, and in hindsight deeply regrettable, progress in understanding the disease was remarkable. In many ways medical advances of the prior 10 years had created a context that allowed the disease to be quickly understood. Initial studies[2] clearly began to show that the disease both was transmitted by sexual contact and had an incubation period during which it still could be spread by asymptomatic carriers. This suggested that the disease might be caused by a virus. Already in the 1950s medical researchers had begun to identify slow or latent viruses that do not have a brief incubation period and rapid onset and resolution. In the past decade there had been considerable work done on retroviruses. Retroviruses are themselves an interesting medical anomaly. Most viruses reproduce by storing their genetic information in DNA. Retroviruses use a process labeled "reverse transcriptase" in which the RNA is transcribed to DNA and then reproduced. By 1983 the responsible virus was identified.[3] This story is in and of itself interesting because it involves monumental egos, national pride, and medical competitiveness. By 1986, an international commission for viral nomenclature labeled the virus HIV (human immunodeficiency virus), ending the confusion between the Pasteur Institute's name LAV (lymphadenopathy associated virus) and U.S. medical researcher Robert Gallo's (1989) preference for the name HTLV III, linking the virus to earlier research that he had done on human T-cell leukemia virus.

At that time, too, the name for the disease was standardized. Initially the disease had generated a number of possible names. Some had suggested GRID—gay-related immune deficiency. This was rejected as both untrue (the disease seemed to spread beyond gay men) and possibly inflammatory. Others suggested CAIDS, community-acquired immune deficiency syndrome, or ACIDS, acquired immune deficiency syndrome. By 1982 the CDC had adopted the name AIDS for acquired immune deficiency syndrome. After 1986, it began to be recognized that AIDS represents the latter stage of HIV infection, sometimes leading to the confusing label HIV/AIDS as many persons in the early stages of HIV infection eschew the label of AIDS.

Researchers also began to recognize how HIV infected and compromised the immune system. The HIV virus seems capable of infecting a number of body cells. But they have their most destructive impact by infecting the T4 cells in the

---

[2]For example, the CDC reports on AIDS from 1981 through 1984 are clear indicators of the gradual understanding emerging about the transmission of HIV/AIDS.

[3]In fact there seem to be two forms of the HIV virus. HIV-1 is the form of virus most commonly found. HIV-2 is a variant found in West Africa. At present both viruses seem to operate in similar ways although there is some suggestion that HIV-2 may be less virulent (Levine, 1992).

immune system. These cells orchestrate attacks on invading microorganisms. By infecting the T4 cells and other cells of the immune system such as B-cells and macrophages, the immune system becomes steadily compromised. Thus the person infected becomes prone to a variety of opportunistic diseases such as PCP, KS, and fungal, bacterial, viral, and other infections and diseases. AIDS, then, is complex. The virus itself may lead to the manifestation of illness, but the most severe effects are likely to arise from other diseases that a compromised immune system can no longer withstand.

THE AIDS PANIC

As knowledge of the disease grew, so did the panic it generated. There were two phases of panic over AIDS. The first phase, 1982–1983, primarily affected risk groups, health professionals, and related service professions. Like earlier epidemic diseases, the panic developed from the fear generated by a new virulent fatal illness with an unknown mode of transmission. And, like earlier epidemics, the behaviors exhibited were both venal and heroic. This phase was characterized by accounts of funeral directors refusing to embalm corpses, medical staff neglecting to treat patients, corrections officers striking in the presence of infected prisoners, and ambulance drivers failing to transport the ill. Heroically, many medical staff fulfilled responsibilities even in the midst of the uncertainty surrounding the disease. Practical actions and behavioral changes also resulted. In response to the condition, the Gay Men's Health Crisis was founded in 1982 to educate, advocate, and provide supportive services to victims and families. And studies indicated that risk groups such as homosexuals did change behaviors (Friedman et al., 1992).

The second phase of the panic in the summer of 1985 was more generalized. Evidence of this phase of panic can be found in a *New York Times* poll of September 12, 1985, in which 51% of the population named AIDS as the most serious disease facing humankind. Manifestations of the panic included widespread reports of discrimination against victims or suspected members of risk groups, calls for quarantines, controversies related to the admission of AIDS-infected students to schools, and over 10,000 calls daily to informational hotlines. Some of the examples from this period demonstrate the degree of panic and hostility the disease generated. For illustration, William F. Buckley, a conservative columnist, called for tattooing persons with AIDS so as to limit their ability to spread the disease. According to Buckley's proposal, addicts would be tattooed in their forearms, gay men on their buttocks.

A particularly heartrending story involved the Ray family in Florida. There, three young boys who were hemophiliacs were all HIV-infected. Not only did the community resist their attending a local school, eventually their house was set afire.

With the panic came various myths. Most of these myths involved deliberate attempts to spread the disease. Shilts (1987), for example, recounts how Gaetan Dugas, one of the first victims of AIDS, had a wanton disregard for the health of others as he continued to have constant, casual, and unsafe sex. Dugas is quoted as telling others after the sexual act, "I've got gay cancer. I'm going to die and so are you." Similarly, Dr. David Acer, a Florida dentist who infected Kimberly Bergalis and five other patients, was accused in an investigative report by Barbara Walters on ABC's *20/20* of infecting these patients deliberately. According to that report, Acer, a gay man dying of AIDS, believed the disease would only get attention if it affected nonstigmatized Americans. Later, other investigative reports would question whether Acer, in fact, infected these patients. These stories, whether true or not, fueled widespread reports and rumors that gay men were deliberately and in large numbers trying to infect other Americans. Meanwhile, many infected persons believed that the disease itself sprang from governmental laboratories, either accidentally or as a conscious plot to eliminate undesirables. Some Black leaders agreed. Louis Farrakan, a Black Muslim leader, saw the disease as a White plot. There was an international dimension as the Soviet KGB planted stories that HIV resulted from U.S. germ warfare efforts.

As stated earlier, Smelser (1963) in his value-laden theory of collective behavior notes three factors necessary for panic. These include structural conduciveness, a precipitating incident, and a mobilization for flight.

The panic observed with AIDS provides a case illustration of Smelser's theory. There were a number of factors contributing to structural conduciveness. The appearance of a virulent fatal disease created anxiety. The disease appeared at a time when many Americans were distrustful of government and established medicine. The very language of science contributed to this underlying ambiguity and anxiety. The language of science is a probabilistic language. Hence, scientifically accurate language that attempted to dismiss fears with tentative, generalized terminology could not provide the certain reassurance that the public demanded. For example, scientific language spoke of "remote possibilities" that AIDS could be spread by tears or saliva. Others persons familiar with the language of science would understand that these probabilities were virtually nonexistent. To the lay population, though, it sounded as if these events could easily happen.

Then, too, the universal medical precautions used with HIV-infected patients seemed to belie medical assurances that the disease was difficult to transmit. As one lay author wrote: "While doctors see AIDS as hard to catch, hospital precautions suggest otherwise" (Lee, 1987, p. 21).

Although it is difficult to point to a single precipitating incident, the accounts of AIDS spreading beyond initial risk groups, as well as reports of more casual modes of transmission (e.g., tears, saliva, insect bites), translated this undercurrent of anxiety into deep fear. Certainly an article published in the prestigious *Journal of the American Medical Association* fueled panic. This article (Oleske et al., 1983) noted the appearance of AIDS in households. Although this would later be recognized as a result of sexual transmission between spouses and prenatal transmission to infants, the authors prematurely and tentatively suggested that AIDS might be spread by casual contact.

In this emerging panic both gay advocacy organizations and the media played a role. There was an assumption on the part of many gay advocacy organizations that the slowness of the response of governmental agencies was a reflection on the perceived social value of the groups at risk. This attitude was well expressed by an editorial in *The Nation*:

> Only one of the many tragic ironies of the AIDS epidemic is that its victims, and those who are at highest risk of infections, have to wait for its spread to more celebrated groups before much progress will be made. . . . Somehow death and disease don't seem as dreadful when they befall other people—especially social groups that may be conveniently blamed for their own misery. ("A Social Disease," 1985, p. 196)

This often led to an emphasis on reports that stressed the seriousness of the health threat by AIDS to the public at large.

It was these reports that were often given the most extensive treatment by the media. As Check (1985) pointed out, it is a misnomer to refer to the media as a single entity, as media encompasses everything from supermarket tabloids to respectable publications to television. Check (1985) noted, however, that the AIDS crisis presented a challenge to the media. First, it was a very complicated story with medical, social, financial, and political dimensions. Second, the complexity of medical research reported in scientific language did not readily translate. Finally, the very competitiveness of the media encouraged a stress on stories that emphasized the spread or increased risk of AIDS.

For example, in 1984–1985, the *New York Times* ran stories of people who did not fall into recognized risk groups: risks to body builders who shared needles in injecting steroids, evidence of AIDS in saliva and tears, testimony regarding the risk of AIDS within the classroom, and reports on transmission through casual contact. Even in its attempts to humanize the disease the media often focused on those it labeled "innocent victims," those like Ryan White who did not develop AIDS due to sexual or drug-related behavior. Although this language of "innocent," and by implication, "deserving," victims is typical of dreaded diseases, particularly sexually transmitted ones such as syphilis, it further stigmatized gays and IV drug users, feeding a belief that only when the disease struck nonmarginalized groups would the country respond.

At the same time, supermarket tabloids claimed that the AIDS virus could be borne in the air, found in water fountains, or transmitted by mosquitoes. As the media reported the fights of various groups (e.g., school boards, etc.), it encouraged and validated similar responses. In short, both groups played a significant role in generating the panic that would impair the treatment of persons with HIV.

THE ORIGIN OF AIDS

Once AIDS was identified in the United States and the West, there was a search to identify the origins of the disease. The search itself was interesting for two reasons. First, it perpetuates a major theme in dreaded diseases—one that associates the disease with others, those on the outside who are responsible for carrying the disease here. The debatable hypothesis that AIDS originated in Africa has interesting parallels with other dreaded diseases. As with those, there is an identification of the disease with sections of the world regarded as less developed. Again there is an image of the disease that is foreign and fearful that stigmatizes those who carry the disease. Second, this concern with origins may obfuscate another critical issue, which is how changing conditions here facilitated the spread of the disease.

This does not deny the fact that there is both scientific and intellectual justification for the origins of a disease. It simply reminds us that we need to recognize how the origins of a disease affect its image, and understand the origins in the context of the larger social conditions.

Initially in the United States, the search began in Haiti. After gay males had emerged as a risk group, other groups were recognized as being at risk. IV drug users and their sexual partners and children began to develop the disease. Persons who had been recipients of blood, particularly hemophiliacs who were treated with Factor VIII, a blood product that used multiple donors, were seen at risk. All of this was logical, supportive of the fact that this disease was spread by some infectious agent, that like hepatitis B, it was transmitted in body fluids such as blood and semen.

But then there were the Haitians. Haitians too were initially identified as a risk group. Recent immigrants from the island seemed to indicate that Haitians were developing the disease at a disproportionate rate. Yet here the logical connection was not obvious. The Haitians involved claimed not to be gay or IV drug users.

This led some to believe that because Haiti had a high incidence of the disease, perhaps it originated there. One theory even suggested that AIDS may be a very old disease. Perhaps, it was a variant of AIDS that Columbus transported to Europe rather than syphilis (Shannon et al., 1991). A contemporary theory conjectured that various voodoo rituals in Haiti that allow the commingling of human and animal blood might have provided opportunities for AIDS-related viruses to develop and then spread to the United States, because Haiti was a mecca for sex tourism among American gay males.

Recent reflection suggests more mundane reasons for the prevalence of AIDS among Haitians. There seems little evidence that AIDS developed in Haiti much before it did in the United States. As Shannon et al. (1991) noted, Haiti was a major source of blood used for blood products and transfusions prior to 1975. If the disease was there early it should have been seen in blood recipients earlier. It is likely that the first victims of AIDS both in Haiti and among Haitian immigrants in the United States were bisexual prostitutes, who would be unlikely to identify themselves as gay because homosexuality is stigmatized so heavily in that culture. The disease then spread by both blood rituals used in voodoo cults, and by an impoverished medical system that reused syringes.

To many, the Haitian connection pointed toward Central Africa. After the tumultuous years of independence, most Belgians abruptly left the Belgian Congo, now Zaire. Their places were often assumed by French-speaking Haitians. Thus it was thought that if the disease did originate in Central Africa it may have then migrated to Haiti before reaching the United States.

There is considerable evidence supporting an African origin of AIDS. Over the past decades a number of new viral diseases such as Lassa, Marburg, and Ebola fevers have emerged from Africa. In fact there is a theory that humans first originated in Africa, but began to migrate elsewhere to escape the plethora of diseases that could emerge in that conducive climate.

There is other evidence as well. The high seropositive rates evident in Africa, particularly in Central Africa, suggest that the disease may have begun there. Then, too, there seems to be a greater variability of strains of HIV, including a major variant HIV-2 that is more prevalent in Western Africa. This suggests greater antiquity. In addition, the earliest cases of AIDS found in Europe had clear African roots. For example, one of the earliest known victims of AIDS in Europe was a Dr. Margaret Rask, a physician who had worked as a surgeon in Zaire. Also, cases of HIV infection have been suspected in Africa as early as 1959, while in the United States the earliest case is a decade later.[4]

The African hypothesis suggests that HIV is related to another virus, SIV (simian immunodeficiency virus). It has been hypothesized that somehow this virus mutated in such a way as to infect humans. Perhaps the mutation was facilitated by a diet of monkeys, bites from monkeys, or rituals that smeared and mixed human and monkey blood. But recent molecular analyses suggest that while this hypothesis is plausible, the truth may be more complex than originally assumed. HIV-2, which was discovered later but did not necessarily originate later than HIV-1, may have been an intermediate step in the evolution of the disease. SIV may have mutated to HIV-2, and then a more virulent HIV-1. Yet correct analysis suggests that while HIV-1 and HIV-2 may share a common ancestor, HIV-1 is the direct descendent of HIV-2. Whether HIV-2 derived from SIV is not yet determined (Mulder, 1988).

Grmek (1990) also notes that the Africa hypothesis is presently unproven. He suggests that AIDS seems almost as recent an occurrence in the West as in Africa. There is also evidence that the disease may have previously existed in the United States, Europe, and especially in South America, particularly in the Amazon.

The origins of a disease have often caused debate and in some cases, such as syphilis, still cause controversy. In the case of HIV/AIDS, this controversy has taken on political overtones. Many Africans have viewed such research to locate the origin of AIDS in Africa as a racially motivated attempt to blame the disease

---

[4]This section draws from Grmek's (1990) excellent study on the origin of AIDS. Grmek offers a careful evaluation of the "African hypothesis," concluding that despite its current popularity it remains unproven.

on others. As in other dreaded diseases there is the assumption that AIDS could not have emerged in the developed world, so it must have its origins in a less developed section. So Africa, Africans, and African practices are blamed for this new plague.

This concern reminds us that the question, "Where did AIDS originate?" is critical. But another critical question is, "Why did AIDS spread at the time that it did?" In order to answer that question, it is important to have some concept of the "when," that is, to know how long the AIDS virus has been around.

Unfortunately there can be no undisputed answer to that question. As with other diseases, we can know when a disease is identified. That does not, however, mean that the disease was not present in more isolated populations, perhaps even populations that managed to coexist with the virus, or that the disease was simply not identified.

Grmek (1990) describes six conditions in which a disease appears to be new. In three of these cases the disease actually is new: the result of a shift in the infectious agent from an animal to a human host, a mutation in the infectious agent that changes its virulence, or the unlikely event of an infectious agent artificially produced either by accident or design. But three other conditions exist as well. In some cases, the disease may have existed in other areas, but becomes new to another region. Or the disease may have escaped medical attention. Finally, the disease may have previously existed but did not appear until there was a qualitative or quantitative change in its manifestations.

It is difficult to pinpoint exactly what factors account for the emergence of AIDS. Certainly it is easier now to detect AIDS. In earlier times, the opportunistic disease itself may have been diagnosed as the cause of illness or death. It is also possible that another disease might have simply escaped notice in the societies of sub-Sahara Africa that have such high death rates. And of course its appearance in the West, as well as a quantitative increase in victims in Africa, led AIDS to be noticed.

It may also be a comparatively new disease. Although there have been some suggestions that AIDS was created either by design or as a by product of the polio vaccination campaign in Africa (e.g., Curtis, 1992), these speculations have little credibility. The prevalent hypotheses see HIV emerging as either a mutation of a virus that may have existed in Africa, perhaps in less virulent forms in an isolated area, or as the previously discussed adaptation from an animal to human host.

The age of the HIV virus has also led to some interesting speculation. Although some, as previously mentioned, see the virus as old, most contemporary researchers see the virus as comparatively new. By calculating the time necessary for the various strains of HIV-1 to emerge, researchers have suggested that the HIV virus has infected humans for at least 20 but not more than 100 years (Grmek, 1990). This time period is reasonably consistent with case reports that sound like HIV infection. The Kaposi's sarcoma epidemic evident in Africa was first noticed in the postwar period. Grmek (1990), in reviewing early suspected cases of HIV/AIDS, finds possible cases as early as the 1950s.

Yet if that were the case, why did the disease seem to emerge only in the late 1970s? An early case is illustrative. One of the first possible U.S. cases was a young, Black, 15-year-old hustler identified as "Robert" who was admitted to the St. Louis Hospital in 1968 and died the following year. The boy seemed to suffer from a variety of opportunistic infections, including Kaposi's sarcoma. Attempts at treatment were unsuccessful because the young man had virtually no immune system. The case so perplexed the doctors that they froze blood and lymph samples for future study. In 1987, medical technology confirmed an underlying diagnosis of HIV infection (Garry et al., 1988).

How and where Robert contracted the HIV virus is unknown. Nor is it known whether or not he transmitted the virus to others. But his case does suggest a possibility. The HIV virus had emerged in the United States at least a decade prior to a major outbreak. It may have surfaced in Europe even earlier. Yet because opportunities for transmitting the virus were limited, it might only have infected a few people before the transmission chain was disrupted. These people died, diagnosed either with an unknown condition or with whatever opportunistic disease struck. In the time they were infected, the disease had limited time to spread. In the 1960s in St. Louis, opportunities for homosexual encounters were limited and somewhat clandestine. Sexual networks then were likely to be small, constraining opportunities for the virus to spread.

However, in the 1970s, conditions became far more conducive to the spread of the virus. In Africa a series of conditions had arisen that both created and increased geographic mobility for the human population and the virus.

The 1970s were a tempestuous and disruptive time in Africa. Part of this disruption was political and military. It was a time of postindependence strife in many countries of Central Africa such as Zaire, Uganda, Burundi, and Rwanda, as well as a time of struggles for independence and civil wars in Angola, Mozambique, Namibia, and Zimbabwe. These wars disrupted African societies, creating waves of refugees fleeing with their diseases. And with the armies came the camp followers.

Second, as Africa began to develop, African men began to migrate into urban areas. In that migrant labor system, wives would often stay in home villages while their men found sexual satisfaction with prostitutes.

Third, as Shannon et al. (1991) pointed out, at this time the Trans-Africa Highway was being built between Mombasa, Kenya, on Africa's west coast to Lagos, Nigeria, in the east. While still incomplete, this highway opened up trade and transport to large sections of Central Africa. As with other diseases, it also allowed the transmission and spread of a virus that may have existed in more isolated areas to larger populations.

If AIDS did originate in Africa, social conditions there in the 1970s were conducive to a much wider spread. Yet it also has to be realized that conditions in other sections of the world such as Europe and the United States also created a context that would be conducive to the spread of this new disease.

One was changing patterns of homosexual activity. Ironically, about a month after Robert, the first confirmed case of AIDS in the United States, died, there was a riot at the Stonewall Bar, a gay bar in New York City. These bars had a tenuous acceptance. They were sometimes tolerated, other times raided by the police. This raid, however, produced a violent riot. To homosexuals, the riot at Stonewall was the opening volley in the struggle for gay liberation. After the riot, the police no longer raided gay bars, and gay culture, at least in larger cities such as San Francisco or New York, could flourish.

The 1970s, then, were a time when gay men and women could openly assert their sexual identity. One observer, Shilts (1987), described the 1970s as a time of sexual experimentation. Long suppressed in a hostile society, gay men entered a phase that Shilts likened to adolescence—sexual activity became a way of show-ing identity and bonding. It was a highly promiscuous era. Studies indicated that many gay men had considerable numbers of sexual encounters, averaging nearly 80–100 (Grmek, 1990).

In some ways, this new era reflected the promiscuity evident in heterosexu-als. But there were factors that institutionalized these patterns of sexual activity that were not evident in the heterosexual world. First, there were few structures encouraging monogamous relationships. Gay relationships lacked any legal standing, sanction, or recognition. Without the legal institution of marriage, there was little incentive to limit sexual activity. Second, there developed within the gay community a variety of settings such as bars and bathhouses that provided opportunities for a wide variety of sexual activity and partners. Although such places existed in the heterosexual world, they were not as widespread. These places were also openly advertised within the gay press. Thus mobile gay men could readily find places for sexual activity as they traveled for business and pleasure. With the increased mobility evident in the 1960s and 1970s there was also increase in tourism, some of which might be called sexual tourism. Some places in the world, such as Thailand, the Philippines, India, and Haiti, became known for providing sexual opportunities. Some of the places provided sexual respite for both heterosexuals and homosexuals.

Because HIV can be spread by certain sexual practices, such as anal intercourse, once the virus was introduced in the gay male population, the possibility of spread became exponential. For example, one French-Canadian airline steward, Gaetan Dugas, in many ways the "Typhoid Mary" or "patient zero" of the AIDS epidemic, reported more than 250 sexual encounters each year. Highly mobile, Dugas facilitated the spread of the disease at least throughout the United States. Long after he was diagnosed with Kaposi's sarcoma, he continued his sexual activity. In a mobile and highly sexual, active gay subculture, the virus could, and did, spread rapidly.

Dugas's story also demonstrates another factor that contributed to the growth of the AIDS epidemic. During the 1970s airline travel for both business and recreational reasons increased dramatically. This provided new opportunities for the disease to spread. In fact, some have called it the "charter disease" (Nord, 1997), reflecting the role that inexpensive airline travel and sexual tourism had in the spread of the disease.

There also were other social changes in the West that facilitated the spread of the disease. Certainly, IV drug use became more common. The late 1960s and the 1970s were a time of increased experimentation with a wide variety of drugs including barbiturates, cocaine, marijuana, hallucinogenic drugs, and amphetamines. Although over time many ceased or minimized drug use, others moved on to drugs such as heroin that were injected. Because the numbers of addicts were higher, a drug subculture, with its own norms and networks, could develop. One behavior that became widespread, at least in some areas, was the sharing of needles. This was considered a friendly act that even transcended the bonding aspect of sharing paraphernalia or a shortage of available equipment. Sharing a needle meant that someone else could get high from the "wash." By filling up a needle with water that mixes with the residues of heroin, one can obtain a high that can hold one until there is an opportunity to buy heroin. Sharing needles would be another vector to spread HIV. In addition, many addicts turned to selling blood or prostitution for money to purchase drugs, providing still more opportunities for the disease to spread.

The selling of blood was another social innovation that occurred in that era and that facilitated the spread of AIDS. The history of blood transfusions may have begun as early as 1490 when a doctor, treating Pope Innocent VIII, attempted to transfuse the blood of three healthy young boys. When all four died, the doctor fled. This treatment counted less on any underlying theory than it did on a general belief that blood was the very fluid of life. But Harvey's work in 1616 on circulation provided the basis of the underlying theory and later work began to identify the uniqueness of human blood, ending fatal experiments transfusing blood between animals and humans. By 1818 a technology for transfusion was developed, but it was Dr. Kay Landsteiner's identification of major human blood groups in 1901 that allowed transfusion to become relatively safe. It was recognized that blood could only be "relatively" safe because certain diseases could be spread through blood.

Once this hurdle was passed blood transfusions became a key therapeutic process used in wide variety of contexts, including operations, accidents, and other situations in which blood was lost. In addition, not only blood, but red blood cells, plasma, and other blood products, were used to treat a variety of diseases and conditions such as anemia and hemophilia.

By the 1960s the demand for blood had greatly intensified. New forms of surgery, especially open heart surgery, and other medical treatment, such as dialysis, helped boost demand. The aging of the population and the concurrent rise in chronic disease as well as new treatments for hemophilia all accentuated the need for human blood. Because donated blood could account for only a small part of that demand, there arose a whole new industry—for-profit blood banks. These centers began in the 1950s but rapidly grew in the 1960s. Titmus (1971) estimates that by the late 1960s they supplied between 30 and 50% of all blood used. Located in some of the poorer sections, they often drew alcoholics and drug addicts as donors. In addition, blood began to be imported, often from poor countries such as Haiti. In discussing the historical development of the commercial blood banks, Titmus (1971) prophetically saw health problems in the development and growth of this new commerce in blood and called for intensive regulation of the blood industry.

The rise of commercial blood centers also became an unwitting vector for the spread of HIV. Commercial blood banks began to emerge as a powerful lobby, controlling a critical commodity and making significant profits. Like other organizations that had commercial interests threatened by AIDS, and other commercial interests in prior dreaded diseases, they were a conservative force, minimizing the possibility of risk and resisting corrective action. For example, blood banks resisted CDC requests to test for antibodies to hepatitis B, a possible and indirect indicator of IV drug use and homosexual activity. Early in the epidemic, many of those infected with HIV had a history of similarly transmitted diseases like hepatitis B (Sapolsky & Boswell, 1992). In addition, the blood industry denied risk and resisted screening donors long after suspicions of transmission of AIDS through transfusion of blood and blood products had been aroused.

While this resistance affected a variety of recipients of donated blood, it deeply threatened persons with hemophilia. In the 1950s, the length and quality of life of patients with hemophilia were dramatically improved by technology that allowed the creation of clotting factors. The most common factors, called Factors VIII and IX, used multiple donors, numbering in the thousands. This meant that hemophiliacs were exposed to the viruses of thousands of donors and that each donor could infect scores of hemophiliacs. By the late 1970s, AIDS was seen in hemophiliacs, but it was not recognized as such until 1982. Because the trade in human blood was now international there were great opportunities for the disease to spread worldwide through the hemophiliac population. Despite the risk, the response of this international blood industry was slow and it was 1985 before significant protective actions were taken. By that point, a majority of hemophiliacs, at least in the United States and other European countries, tested positive for HIV.

In summary, while the HIV virus likely existed for a period of time prior to the 1970s, it probably only infected isolated groups of people. Significant social changes in the 1970s—changes in patterns of mobility as well as in sexual behaviors, drug use, and blood use and collection—created a context in which a viral disease such as HIV/AIDS could rapidly spread. Whenever human behavior undergoes significant changes, the relationships between humans and their parasites undergoes modification as well. New patterns of mortality replace older patterns.

Since emerging in the 1970s, the AIDS pandemic has demonstrated distinct patterns in different parts of the world. In Western Europe, North America, Australia, New Zealand, and urban areas of Latin America, the disease primarily infects gay men, IV drug users, and persons infected through blood products. Heterosexual and perinatal transmission represent a small but increasing proportion of those infected. In sub-Sahara Africa, parts of Latin America, and the Caribbean, HIV was recognized about the same time, but it primarily spread through heterosexual intercourse and use of blood and unsterile needles. Perinatal transmission is more common in these areas because both genders are affected equally. In Eastern Europe, the Middle East, North Africa, Asia, and the Pacific the disease is beginning to emerge among those engaged in high-risk behaviors. While the World Health Organization originally used to designate areas as exhibiting a distinctive pattern, it is becoming increasingly recognized that the HIV/AIDS pandemic is highly dynamic, unstable, and still rapidly spreading to areas of the world where it was previously unrecognized.

CONCLUSION

Once AIDS became recognized, it rapidly emerged as a dreaded disease. In many ways, AIDS represents the archetype of the dreaded diseases, combining the factors that made previous diseases, described in earlier chapters, so feared.

What is it about AIDS that we fear? Everything. Like the crises of contagion, it is both virulent and mysterious. Its continual geometric spread and its early incorporation of new risk groups terrified the populace. Its long incubation period and comparatively common initial symptoms heightened anxiety. Until the development of the AIDS test in 1987, there was little way to assess whether these rather generic early symptoms such as night sweats or diarrhea might be harbingers of AIDS. Prior to 1983, its method of transmission was itself mysterious. Even now we do not fully understand why some infected individuals rapidly develop full-blown AIDS while others show a slower progression of HIV infection. As in other epidemics, there was often an interpretation by some religious figures, such as Jerry Falwell, that the "Gay Plague" was divine retribution.[5]

AIDS also shares the characteristics of the stigmatizing diseases. It is chronic, painful, invariably fatal, disfiguring, and debilitating. AIDS associates sex, sin, deviance, and death. As a *National Review* editorial proclaimed, "AIDS remains a permanent skeleton at the feast of sexual liberation." Thus, not only is the disease stigmatizing in itself, but it carries a "double jeopardy." The victim is identified with socially defined deviant groups such as homosexuals or drug addicts. Hence the disease carries a strong moral connotation in which victims are blamed for their fate. This is evident in columnist Ray Kerison's (1985) comment on AIDS victim Victor Bender's testimony before a congressional committee:

---

[5]A position vigorously refuted by other religious figures.

"With all due deference to the man's suffering it bothers me when he lashes out at public officials without anywhere accepting personal responsibility for his own actions or lifestyle" (p. 4).

As Sontag (1978) noted:

> Nothing is more punitive than to give disease a meaning—that meaning invariably a moral one. Any important disease whose causality is murky and for which treatment is ineffectual tends to be awash in significance. First, the subjects of deepest dread (corruption, decay, pollution, anomie, weakness) are identified with the disease. The disease itself becomes a metaphor. Then, in the name of that disease (that is, using as a metaphor), the horror is imposed on other things. The disease itself becomes adjectival, meaning that it is disgusting or ugly. (p. 58)

The nature of AIDS itself has become the metaphor that Sontag warned against, a metaphor that strikes at the fears of a complex society—death from systemic breakdown, invasion, and decay.

In addition, AIDS is spread through blood and semen, fluids of life, often historically invested with mystical significance. Frazier (1922) in his classic work *The Golden Bough* noted the universal prevalence of the significance of blood. To Frazier blood has always had a mystical significance because it was often believed that the soul or spirit resided in the blood. Hence blood was used in rituals of purification, community, and magic, to connote long-lasting "blood" feuds, or to secure covenants and lasting friendships. Thus a disease that is spread through blood and other fluids associated with the powers of life strikes a deep, almost primal fear. This is especially true when the disease mixes blood, death, and sex. Wolf (1972) pointed out that vampire legends exist in many different parts of the world. He further explores the connections between blood, sex, and death. In the Dracula legend, for example, the vampire drains life through a passionate blood kiss. AIDS is the new vampire—the kiss that kills.

As the horror of cancer, the dreaded disease of earlier decades, has subsided due to effective treatment, AIDS has moved to take its place. If some demonic mind wished to devise a new dreaded disease, he or she could not have done better than AIDS. Not only does AIDS combine many of the characteristics of other dreaded diseases, it also is intertwined with marginality, morality, and metaphor, and rooted in an almost primal awe of the fluids of life—blood and semen. The effect of this fear, while discussed earlier, will also be explored in a subsequent chapter.

Chapter 5

PROMISES AND PROBLEMS: THE MEDICAL ENCOUNTER WITH AIDS

It is time to close the book on infectious diseases.
Surgeon General W. H. Stewart, 1969

Even without motivation, it is always possible that some hitherto obscure parasite organism may escape its accustomed ecological niche and expose the dense human populations . . . to some fresh and perchance devastating mortality.
McNeill, Plagues and Peoples

McNeill's statement almost seems prophetic two decades later. As his book was published, a new parasitic virus was about to devastate humankind.

It is the impact of that encounter that will be explored in subsequent chapters. But prior to that, it is critical to explore medicine's encounter with this new disease. For the future of this disease will be far different if an effective cure, treatment, vaccine, or strategy for prevention emerges. The thesis of this chapter is that prevention is limited, and an effective vaccine or cure is remote. The prospect of more effective treatment holds considerable promise, but paradoxically creates additional problems.

As discussed in earlier chapters, the initial medical encounter with HIV/ AIDS was twofold. On one hand, there was an unpreparedness for the encounter with a new infectious disease that bordered on medical arrogance. Despite numerous encounters with new viral diseases such as Marburg fever, there was only a slow recognition that a new viral disease was spreading throughout the world. Again part of this arrogance was a neglect to view the health problems of the third world, where epidemics had historically begun as a possible threat to more developed countries. Had the African "wasting" disease, as AIDS was called there, been identified and researched, the epidemic's spread might have been slowed. Yet even here the pervasive spread of HIV into areas that it had not yet entered early in the epidemic, such as Asia, suggest that such hope may be misplaced.

Once science was mobilized, its progress was surprisingly fast. Based upon the pioneering work done in the previous decade on retroviruses, the HIV virus was quickly identified and the process of infection and viral reproduction generally understood. Tests identifying the presence of antibodies to the virus were also rapidly produced allowing science both to trace the disease's spread and to begin early treatment. Treatments also were developed that gradually extended the life of those infected with the virus.

AIDS AS A SYNDROME:
THE NATURE OF THE DISEASE

One of the first lessons learned, and in a sense, one that is still ongoing, is about the nature of AIDS as a disease. Actually, AIDS may be said to be both a disease and a syndrome. By that it is meant that the HIV virus directly infects the immune system, as well as cells, and by doing so increases the susceptibility of the body to opportunistic diseases and neoplasms.

Specifically the HIV virus most directly attracts the CD4 receptors of T lymphocytes. These cells are critical to the body's immune functions. T lymphocytes, or T-cells as they are commonly known, are the body's first line of defense against infection. In addition to T-cells, the virus also attacks monocytes (when these cells enter tissues from the bloodstream, they are called macrophages). These, too, are critical to the body's defense, serving a number of functions— some still not fully understood—that include assisting in identifying foreign matter, digesting foreign matter, and producing antimicrobial and antiviral substances. The HIV virus can also attack specific cells of the gastrointestinal tract (called glial cells) and the central nervous system, and other cells such as uterine cervical cells.

Some people, perhaps 10–15% of those infected, have an acute retroviral reaction evidenced in flu or mononucleosis-like symptoms such as a fever or rash (F. Cohen, 1995). This seems to occur anywhere between 5 days to 3 months after the infection, though in most cases it is between 2 and 4 weeks. In this early period, the body produces antibodies that are detected in the most common HIV tests such as the enzyme-linked immunosorbent assay (ELISA) and Western blot tests. However, it is important to realize that for anywhere up to 6 weeks, these antibodies may not be present. This means there is a window where the infected person may still test negative for HIV infection.

Whether or not this acute retroviral reaction occurs, most persons enter a long period in which they are relatively asymptomatic; that is, they test positive for HIV infection but show no symptoms of disease or even, in the early period of this asymptomatic phase, signs of immune impairment. It was once thought that HIV was in this early period relatively dormant or contained by the body's immune system. Recent evidence suggests otherwise. Ho et al. (1995) have presented evidence that suggests the immune system and HIV are engaged in a pitched battle from the time of infection. Millions of viruses are killed daily by the immune system, which itself must replace almost a billion infected and dying cells. Basically, Ho et al. (1995) suggested that HIV infection is like an acute infection that never ends. In time the gradual imbalance shifts to the virus's favor. More and more viruses are produced, overwhelming the immune system. The research of Ho et al. (1995) offers both good and bad news for treatment. The good news is that it suggests that anti-HIV drugs can often kill a large percentage of the virus, giving the immune system more time to mount a response. The bad news is that the virus's ability to mutate often makes it quickly resistant to drugs.

As the immune system becomes impaired, the body is less able to resist opportunistic infections and neoplasms. First there may be early signs of a weakened immune system such as generalized and persistent lymphadenopathy or various fungal infections such as oral candidiasis (thrush), continued fevers, and night sweats. The person may also experience varied opportunistic diseases such as *Pneumocystis carinii* pneumonia (PCP), toxoplasmosis (caused by the herpes virus), tuberculosis, and cryptococcal meningitis (a fungal disease), among others. These diseases are called opportunistic because most people with healthy immune systems would have little difficulty in fighting them. Infected persons also have an increased susceptibility to neoplasms such as Kaposi's sarcoma (an aggressive skin cancer) and lymphomas.

HIV is considered a progressive disease. Over the years, Walter Reed Hospital and the Centers for Disease Control and Prevention have developed various forms of classification of the disease based on symptomatology and CD4 cell counts. However, much like the earlier classifications of ARC (AIDS-related complex) and AIDS, these have limited value. For example, even persons still not classified as having the latter stage of the disease, now popularly known as AIDS, which is evidenced by the presence of certain opportunistic diseases and neoplasms, may still be quite sick and debilitated, sometimes even more than those with full-blown AIDS. More recent tests that allow measurement of the actual presence of the virus in the blood—the "viral load"—will undoubtedly lead to different ways of conceptualizing the progression and course of the disease.

This is one of the reasons that HIV infection is really a syndrome. The course of the disease can be highly individual. Each infected individual may have a different range of opportunistic diseases, neoplasms, and other conditions affecting different bodily systems, causing unique sets of symptoms and mandating varied treatments. For example, some may experience dementia, as a result of either direct central nervous system infection or other conditions such as herpes. Various psychiatric manifestations, such as depression, anxiety disorders, mania, and delirium, also may be evident in AIDS; these disorders may be a direct result of HIV infection or a reaction to the HIV infection (Winiarski, 1991). Some may be blinded by cytomegalovirus (CMV). Others may exhibit a wasting syndrome. And different risk groups such as infected children and IV drug users, as well as groups in different areas, may exhibit varied manifestations of the disease. For example, infected children often show a failure to thrive, chronic nasal discharge, chronic and persistent diarrhea, oral candidiasis (thrush), and *Candida dermatitis* (diaper rash) that is unresponsive to treatment. In Africa, the wasting or "slim disease" and Kaposi's sarcoma are common, while PCP is not as prevalent. The syndrome may be different in men and women. In women, for example, Kaposi's sarcoma is not as common. Instead, women may be infected with other conditions such as pelvic inflammatory disease and vaginal fungal infections.

In summary, then, HIV is an exceedingly complex syndrome that directly infects certain cells, including immune cells. By weakening the immune system, the virus indirectly allows other opportunistic infections and neoplasms to attack the host. These indirect effects are so individual that the course and time of the disease can vary widely from one person to another. And it is these indirect effects that will eventually kill the infected person.

CONTROLLING THE FUTURE

But what can be expected of the future? The future course of the disease will depend on the ability to prevent the disease through education and lifestyle changes and the development of a vaccine, cure, or improved treatment. The hope of prevention through education and lifestyle changes is at least somewhat illusory. In theory HIV infection is totally preventable because it is not insect-borne or spread through casual contact. If no new cases of HIV infection developed, the disease would die out for lack of hosts in less than two decades.

Yet that is unlikely to occur. First, there is the argument from history. Other sexually transmitted diseases have continued to infect the population for hundreds of years. Syphilis, in particular, should have been eradicated. After all, it is spread in ways even more limited than AIDS. Infection can also be determined through medical testing. Syphilis can even be cured. Still the disease has proved surprisingly resilient.

The nature of HIV infection also inhibits prevention. HIV has a long asymptomatic period. During this time neither the carriers nor their partners may be aware of the risk of infection. Then, too, even when it develops the disease can lack clear outward identifying signs that can warn others of potential risk.

The fact that the disease is transmitted primarily through unsterile needles or sexual contact also troubles prevention. Sex is a pleasurable, drive-based behavior that is hard to control by rational appeals. IV drug use is an addictive behavior. And in many third world countries, sterilization of syringes is considered a luxury.

There is also the geography of the disease. The epicenters of the disease in the third world are among some of the poorest nations in the world. Torn by conflict, many of these nations lack a basic infrastructure, inhibiting a response to the disease. Culture and economics constrain the use of condoms or sterilized needles. Cultural practices such as scarification may contribute to the disease. Continued political and social turmoil and the movements of refugees and armies provide new opportunities for the disease to spread. Suspicion of the medical institution and the West and low rates of literacy create barriers to prevention.

In the West, similar constraints are present. Many of those infected with HIV are marginalized members of society. Persons of color may have a great suspicion of the government and the medical establishment. As mentioned earlier in this book, in the United States the Tuskegee experiments have contributed to a legacy of distrust. In fact, there is often an underlying suspicion that the disease itself is being purposely spread by the government. In many cultures, abortion or the use of condoms are disdained. Low literacy rates inhibit prevention through education.

The gay community, which has suffered through stigma and discrimination, tends to view the government and medical establishment with similar suspicion, viewing them as indifferent at best, and at worst willfully engaging in genocide. The message of AIDS prevention sharply contrasts with one of the tenets of post-Stonewall gay life, sexual liberation.

In Western society as a whole, particularly in the United States, there is still a reluctance to seriously address issues of drug use or sexuality, especially homosexuality, in a realistic and frank way. This mutes the message of prevention. For example, many U.S. television networks still prohibit advertisements on the use of condoms.

Although the incidence of new cases of HIV infection within the United States and other developed countries has leveled off somewhat, the disease continues to spread elsewhere. Even more frightening is the fact that HIV has spread to new areas that previously had low rates of HIV infection. Cases of HIV infection, for example, have rapidly increased in southeast Asia even though these societies had more than a decade to attempt to forestall an epidemic. Clearly prevention alone cannot halt the epidemic.

Prevention and Testing

Prevention will work best if persons, at least those at risk for the disease, are aware of their HIV status and act accordingly. Since 1985, tests have been available that show the presence of antibodies for HIV. Together the two most common tests, the ELISA and Western blot tests, offer a high degree of accuracy (McDonal et al., 1989). More recently developed tests, such as the polymerase chain reaction tests, that directly measure the presence of HIV are likely to become more important in the future, particularly if a vaccine is produced, because someone vaccinated will show antibodies.

Subsequent chapters will explore aspects of HIV tests from historical, political, and counseling perspectives. Testing will have a limited role in prevention. In many cases, individuals may not know their status. And that status may change over time. In addition, even individuals who know they are infected may not modify behaviors simply as a result of that knowledge. For example, IV drug users may still share needles. There are many compelling psychosocial reasons to have children. It does not necessarily follow that individuals who know they are infected will not become pregnant. Although Cuba has instituted mandatory testing with quarantines of infected individuals, it is still unclear how effective such an approach will be. And in many Western societies, at least, such actions would seriously violate concepts of civil liberties. Despite these difficulties, testing for HIV infection will have to be, along with education, part of a preventive program.

Vaccines

Vaccines have been a promising prospect for control. Historically vaccines have been the great success in the war on viruses. Vaccines have eradicated smallpox and seem well on their way to eliminating polio and measles. In fact, as soon as researchers confirmed that AIDS was caused by a virus, there was a sense that a vaccine might be developed within the decade.

Now much of that optimism has dissipated. As we have learned more about the IIIV virus it has become increasingly clear that it has many tricks to defend itself. By infecting the CD4 cells, HIV inhibits an effective response.

But even more problematic is the fact that HIV is genetically unstable. Like the influenza virus, it changes into so many different strains. The protection yielded by one strain may be highly limited. This also raises additional practical problems should the vaccine be made from strains prevalent in the given area.

Past vaccines have essentially been crude. Using killed or weakened viruses, these vaccines worked by triggering a massive pouring of antibodies that conferred lasting immunity. Yet this does not seem possible with AIDS. First, the ability of the body's antibodies to forestall infection seems limited. Second, given the instability of the virus, utilizing a weakened virus seems dangerous. It is even possible that if enough of the viral material were present, it could evolve and infect the cell. Even if the weakened virus did not infect a cell, there might be other problems. Retroviruses are able to manipulate genes. The long-term effect of such a virus, introduced in a vaccine, is unclear. Some believe that it might be carcinogenic.

As mentioned earlier in this book, another strategy that has been suggested for the AIDS vaccine is using "recombinant" technology, which is part of the successful hepatitis B vaccine. Here a small piece of the viral protein is introduced to generate antibodies. This strategy, though seemingly safe, has had mixed results in field tests. Given the demography of HIV infection, complicated vaccine regimens involving multiple vaccines and periodic boosters are unlikely to be effective. Then, too, if such an approach is attempted, there is the question of which proteins may be most stable and effective in an essentially unstable virus.

Beyond the questions, there are practical problems. Who should receive the vaccine? Given the risk of any vaccine, especially the potentially heightened risk of an HIV vaccine, this is a critical question. With diseases such as smallpox or polio, it was clear that the largest possible population should be inoculated. These diseases put anyone at risk. The dangers inherent in any vaccination seemed a small price to pay. With HIV, however, not everyone is at risk. Perhaps the vaccine should be offered primarily to populations at risk, as was done with the hepatitis B vaccine. Yet for the hepatitis B vaccine, inoculation is most widespread in health care workers rather than populations such as IV drug users where the risk is greater. In the West, the stigma associated with IV drug use or homosexuality could discourage possible candidates. Then, too, if the vaccine is developed, it may be counterproductive, encouraging persons to resume high-risk activities, even though protection is incomplete. And certainly there are political issues to overcome. In the United States the active participation of affected communities will be essential to test a vaccine. Yet within the affected communities, there is suspicion of the government and medical establishment and a lack of consensus on the value of a vaccine. Some believe that monies would best be spent on treatment, and others feel that vaccines would encourage continued risky behaviors.

Despite the millions that the U.S. Public Health Service has spent on finding a vaccine, there is a continuing sense of skepticism about a vaccine's possible effectiveness. Yet the incentive for a vaccine is still there. Given the limits to curing HIV, the best strategy still seems to be to inhibit initial infection. Even a vaccine with a comparatively low rate of protection might forestall the spread of HIV, assuming, of course, that individuals vaccinated did not carelessly engage in risky behaviors. Experience with syphilis has shown that the successful treatment led to increases in risky behaviors. Vaccines, along with microbicides or other drugs that could neutralize the virus at a point of entry, seem ways to control the disease. Yet they could lead to an increase in risky behaviors. But vaccines, unfortunately, will not be so easily or so accidentally developed as in the past. Hope even for a limited vaccine still remains. Since 1995, the World Health Organization has been conducting large trials of an AIDS vaccine. But skepticism still remains. The United States rejected requests to participate in that trial because there were serious questions about the vaccine's effectiveness.

Cure and Treatment

The hope of a cure is rarely mentioned in HIV research. The reason is clear. Science has really not found a way to kill viruses once they have infected a host. An antiviral cure for HIV would be the ultimate medical long shot. It would be the equivalent of the discovery of penicillin, an antibiotic capable of killing a wide variety of bacterial infections. We would have to be that lucky once again to discover an antiviral drug as effective as penicillin has been against bacteria.

Primarily the strategies against viruses have been threefold. First, there are strategies that seek to control or minimize symptoms until the immune system can eliminate the virus. That is essentially the value of cold medications. They minimize the symptoms of a cold while the immune system eventually kills the virus. A second strategy involves bolstering the immune system to enhance its defensive functions. For example, gamma globulin is sometimes used to bolster immune systems so they can more efficiently fight disease. A third strategy is to use drugs that inhibit the reproduction of viruses. This makes it easier for the immune system to mobilize against the virus.

All of these strategies are utilized in some degree within both conventional and nonconventional therapies for HIV infection. At present, conventional treatment for HIV infection has been fourfold. First, there are therapies aimed at directly attacking or inhibiting the HIV virus. These therapies include such drugs as zidovudine (AZT), didanosine, and dideoxycytidine. Second, there are therapies that seek to enhance the immune system so it can be more effective in sustaining itself and fighting HIV infection. These therapies can include a variety of strategies such as immune enhancement, which seeks through interferon or interleukin-2 to increase the effectiveness of the immune system and stimulate a more aggressive response, and immunotherapy, which attempts to rebound the immune system through bone marrow transplant or the administration of immune system elements such as globulins or white blood cells. Third, there are therapies that seek to prevent or treat opportunistic diseases. Finally, there are therapies directed against neoplasms. These include chemotherapy, radiation, surgery, and in some cases immunotherapy. Yet all are of limited use because they all ultimately depend on the immune system to destroy the virus. The insidiousness of HIV lies in the fact that it is the immune system that is under attack. Treatment cannot eliminate the infected cells because this would destroy the CD4 cells. Such a process would leave the body as defenseless as it would be in full-blown AIDS.

Because a vaccine or cure is considered unlikely, much attention has been placed on the issue of control. It is beyond the scope of this book to fully describe the varieties of conventional and alternative therapies that now exist to treat persons infected with HIV. Rather, this section develops three critical theses. First, the treatment of HIV has shown considerable progress in the past decade. Second, the HIV infection is extraordinarily complex. Finally, the success and complexity of treatment have considerable implications for health care and prevention.

The ability of medicine to develop treatments for HIV infection is remarkable. In little more than a decade, the virus was identified and treatment was established. A number of strategies have proved somewhat effective. Perhaps the greatest success has been in treating opportunistic diseases that resulted from the weakened immune system. For example, early in the epidemic, PCP was often fatal. Now a variety of drugs such as Bactrim or pentamidine have been developed to successfully treat the disease. This progress in treating these opportunistic diseases has contributed much to the enhanced survival rate of persons with HIV.

Less success has been achieved with drugs that attempt to slow or kill HIV directly. Zidovudine, formally called AZT or azidothymidine, was found to be effective in delaying opportunistic infections in asymptomatic patients. Zidovudine works by inhibiting retroviral reverse transcriptase. In addition, there are two other available reverse transcriptase inhibitors, didanosine and dideoxycytidine, which can be used with zidovudine in a combination therapy. Here the virus's ability to mutate seems to make such drugs less effective over the long run (Ho et al., 1995).

Yet in 1996, even more positive therapies were developed. In addition to reverse transcriptase inhibitors, a new class of drugs, protease blockers, were developed. Such drugs—ritonavir and indinavir (with more on the way)—block the activity of HIV protease, an enzyme of the HIV virus. Such action also blocks the reproductive cycle of the HIV virus. In addition to these new weapons, current strategies stress using multiple drugs—both blockers and inhibitors—in combination, because this makes it much more difficult for the virus to mutate in a way that allows it to become resistant to all the drugs currently employed against it. And by limiting the reproduction of the virus, fewer viruses are produced, reducing the odds for a successful mutation. Although these results are positive, it is still premature and dangerous to tout the end of the plague (Sullivan, 1996). The long-term ability of these strategies to control the HIV virus is untested. In addition, both the cost and difficulty of adhering to a complex drug regimen inhibit wide usage. And such premature calls could encourage increases in risky behaviors.

The treatment of HIV remains highly complex. There are a number of reasons for this. First, there is considerable disagreement about when drugs should be used. Most of these treatments have toxic side effects, some quite serious. Zidovudine, the presently most successful therapy, has had mixed results. Some studies have found that early antiretroviral treatment slowed the progression of the disease, but other studies found it neither slowed the progression of disease nor enhanced survival time compared with those who deferred treatment. It is clear that zidovudine's effectiveness seems to be reduced over time, suggesting that combination treatments alternating antiretroviral therapies may be most effective. Such a regimen is effective for a number of reasons. Not only do multiple combinations of therapies reduce viral resistances, but they may also simultaneously attack multiple sites in the replication cycle and reduce toxic side effects. Yet there is a clear lack of consensus on when it is appropriate to begin therapies or protocols for combining therapies. This lack of consensus, as well as the unpredictability of the disease, makes it very confusing for patients and physicians alike. For example, a recent study suggested that interleukin-2, an immune enhancer, is effective in increasing the proliferation of T-cells in patients with a CD4 count of 200+ CD4 cells mm/L. However, in patients with counts less than that, it seemed to lead to increased viral activation, few immunological improvements, and significant toxic side effects (Kovacs et al., 1995). This suggests the complexity of treating HIV because some treatments may have very different effects at various points in the illness. The fact that some medical researchers suggest that early treatments may be limited to medications aimed at preventing certain conditions such as PCP confuses the issue further.

Second, these regimens are expensive and require significant medical monitoring because the course of the disease is quite variable in individuals and many of the therapies have toxic side effects. In addition, many of them have been primarily tested on gay and bisexual males because they have been a generally available and cooperative population. But this makes the results problematic to apply to other populations, especially women, infected with HIV. And all of these factors complicate the effective use of such therapies in the third world or with populations such as IV drug users who are likely to be less than conscientious in adhering to a complicated medical regimen. Adherence to treatment usually involves a number of factors, including the nature of the treatment itself. Protocols involving medications that are orally administered, convenient to take, comparably inexpensive, and have minimum toxicity or side effects are more likely to be adhered to or followed. Current HIV treatment does not meet these conditions. In addition, adherence is affected by characteristics of the person following treatments. Persons in unstable situations or dealing with multiple problems are less likely to adhere to a treatment. This is especially true with the new, quite promising combination therapy. Here, the treatment regimen is quite complex: It involves taking a variety of pills, at precise times, under specific conditions (e.g., on an empty stomach). Failure to follow the regimen can be quite detrimental, perhaps breeding new, resistant strains of the virus. Currently, in determining whether to use the therapy, physicians must evaluate how likely a candidate is to be compliant. And the regimen is very expensive, currently costing $15,000 a year.

Finally, these treatments, like those for cancer, coexist with a wide range of alternative therapies. Some of these, such as holistic approaches of massage, nutrition, imaging, and visualization, may be more adequately termed complimentary therapies—they can be done in addition to conventional medical treatment. They are unlikely to interfere with treatment and may be beneficial for a number of reasons, not the least being that the person believes in the approach and experiences a renewed sense of control.

But like the cancer underground, there exists, in the United States and elsewhere in the West, a considerable underground in HIV medication. Part of this underground includes "private drug research." A small number of physicians, primarily in New York or San Francisco, have treated patients outside of FDA-approved clinical trials testing new medications. For example, in San Francisco, Project Inform tested a compound Q, made from a Chinese cucumber. This only became known after some patients had died. This underground also tries to facilitate the use of drugs, many experimental, that have not yet been approved or are available only in other countries. The FDA's approval of a parallel track that allows physicians to provide experimental medications in certain circumstances to those not enrolled in clinical trials was given in part to minimize the motivations for alternative therapies. Yet as the continued resilience of the alternative therapies in cancer indicate, this is likely to be only partially successful. There are a number of reasons for this. First, many persons infected with HIV are educated and articulate. They are able to be active participants in treatment, informed of advantages and disadvantages of various therapies, especially conventional ones. Second, they are a desperate population, with little to lose. Third, there is an activist network among persons with HIV providing opportunities for alternative therapies to be shared. Fourth, much of the infected population, as members of groups that have experienced societal stigma and discrimination, distrust governmental and medical agencies. Finally, many alternative physicians have been described as more open to providing emotional support to persons with HIV and incorporating them as participants in treatment. Thus the AIDS underground is likely to be as long-lasting as the disease.

The fact that control through treatment rather than cure is likely to remain the most effective strategy for confronting the HIV epidemic has three major implications. First, as mentioned earlier, it is likely to make the experience of the disease considerably different in developing nations than it is in developed nations. In developing nations, the complicated regimen of treatment and its expense will limit all but rudimentary and primitive treatment to few persons, essentially in the urban elite. It can be expected, then, that while survival time increases in the Western industrialized nations, it will probably only show minimal increases in developing countries.

But this raises two other implications. The cost of HIV treatment will become a major cost to health care in the United States and in other Western nations. In the United States particularly, the HIV epidemic is likely to significantly modify the health care system. The treatment of HIV is expensive, and many persons infected with HIV may lack adequate private coverage or fail to qualify for Medicaid. In any case, the ongoing care of persons with the disease will add significant costs to health care.

In addition, as in syphilis, the very nature of the disease creates ideal conditions for its continued spread. HIV infection is a chronic disease in which the virus can be transmitted at any point in the illness. The disease also has a long asymptomatic period during which neither the infected person nor prospective partners may be aware of infection. Even in the later course of the disease, many symptoms of AIDS are not readily distinguishable from other conditions, again providing little warning of infection that could inhibit transmission. Effective treatment may extend survival time and increase the amounts of time that an individual is generally well and asymptomatic. This in turn provides additional opportunities for the disease to spread to others. Because the behaviors that spread HIV in the West are need-driven—IV drug use and sexual behaviors— treatment has to be combined with strategies for education and prevention.

CONCLUSION

Despite hopes for an effective vaccine or cure for AIDS, it seems that people will have to live in a world in which HIV is part. HIV is too imbedded in the population to simply disappear. Sexually transmitted diseases historically have been difficult to eradicate even under the best of circumstances.

There is a curious process of adaptation between microbes and their hosts. Over time, the less virulent forms are the ones most likely to reproduce and spread. Parasites that too quickly weaken or kill their hosts are less likely to spread. In the evaluation of parasite organisms, the survival of the fittest still holds. But in the complex dance between parasite and host, the most benign parasites are the fittest.

Syphilis became a less virulent disease in the space of about 150 years. With HIV, such a process is likely to be slower. HIV is already reasonably well adapted to its host. It gives few clues of initial infection, has a long, asymptomatic latency period, and very slowly debilitates its host.

Ironically, some have suggested that one strategy of fighting this disease might be to help the host become more adaptive to the virus. Dr. Geoffrey Hoffman, a University of British Columbia immunologist, in a complex and unconventional approach, essentially believes that HIV creates an intense autoimmune reaction, that is, that HIV triggers an immune system attack on a variety of cells within the host (Kion & Hoffman, 1991). Hoffman's solution is an "antivaccine"— a vaccine that makes the body tolerate rather than resist the virus. At present, Hoffman's work has generated interest but little support. It is still considered very theoretical and tentative at best.

If anything at all, HIV should remind society of the possibility that it is simply a harbinger of other new possible diseases. A constant theme of this book is that ecology reminds society that when one organism is removed from a niche, other organisms will have new opportunities to fill that role. As humans conquer viral diseases, those very conquests may provide openings for other viruses heretofore unknown. And sociology reinforces the idea that as societies and patterns of interaction change, and the pace of those changes is now very rapid, each change disturbs the very tenuous balance of nature.

Chapter 6

POLICIES, POLITICS, AND PUBLIC HEALTH

AIDS is treated more like a civil rights issue that has implications for public health than a public health issue that has implications for civil rights.

Anonymous

Similar to past dreaded diseases, AIDS is a threat to both public health and civil liberties and the social order. The AIDS epidemic could lead to significant disruptions in society as well as curtailments of civil rights and other restrictions on human behaviors. As in the past, threats to public health can create tensions between individual and societal rights.

HIV/AIDS has been a contentious issue, spawning debates on effective strategies for prevention as well as conflicts over discrimination, access to health care, and confidentiality. At the heart of all these debates is essentially the issue of balancing the rights of the infected, the uninfected, and the society at large. As in other dreaded diseases, these debates have often been politically polarized.

This chapter reviews and reflects on the ways that these debates have become politicized. It explores the thesis that the politization of AIDS has been a major impediment to the development of effective policies to lessen the threat to public health.

PERSPECTIVES FROM THE PAST

Previous encounters with dreaded diseases have often led to significant restrictions on civil liberties. Past actions to control feared and dreaded diseases were often draconian. Persons with the disease were quarantined or even driven away. Public health responses to such diverse dreaded diseases as tuberculosis, leprosy, and polio generally included quarantines or segregation in specialized facilities either on a voluntary or involuntary basis. Individuals such as Typhoid Mary who resisted restrictions were often dealt with severely. Discrimination was ignored or even encouraged. Few questioned institutions, even health care institutions. During the polio epidemic, public health officials in New York and other cities routinely conducted house-to-house searches. And in World War I, more than 18,000 accused prostitutes were detained and tested for syphilis. Even the general population tended to acquiesce to curtailments of their own freedoms or opportunities, whether it be a requirement, as in the influenza epidemic, that persons wear masks or widespread closings of public facilities and curtailment of services, as in the polio and cholera epidemics. Often there was little respect for notions of confidentiality. Many states in the United States, for example, mandated tests for syphilis as a precondition for marriage and some mandated contact tracing.

CURRENT RESPONSES
TO THE HIV/AIDS EPIDEMIC

The Cuban Response

Some of the abovementioned policies have been implemented in the HIV/AIDS epidemic. Cuba's response has been one of the most severe. In some ways, Cuba was as much at risk for the disease as Haiti. Many of its soldiers and civilians had served in the African equatorial belt, particularly Angola and Mozambique where AIDS was rampant. Recognizing the possible threat, Cuban health officials instituted two major thrusts. First, they began mass, mandatory testing of the population. By 1991 the Cuban Ministry of Public Health reported that more than 35% of the population aged 15 years and older had been tested (Perez-Stable, 1991). Even more controversial was their second action. Those who tested positive were quarantined in one of six rural, remote facilities, an action that had no earlier precedent or legal basis in the Cuban Constitution.

The Cuban Ministry of Health claims the program has been highly success-ful. Their own reports show an extremely low rate of seroprevalence (0.00009%) (Perez-Stable, 1991). Yet others question those claims. Certainly studies of persons who entered the United States in the Mariel boatlift had a much higher sero-prevalence (approximately 0.4%), though this may reflect a selected population. In addition, the claims of the Cuban Ministry may have to be taken with a grain of salt. As in other Communist, or formally Communist countries such as Romania, AIDS presents an ideological challenge. Behaviors that constitute possible risk factors such as homosexuality or IV drug use are often considered capitalist vices that do not exist in the socialist state. For example, it is Cuba's position that IV drug use has been eliminated: "The MINSAP [Cuban Ministry of Public Health] cate-gorically states that illicit intravenous drug use does not exist in Cuba and thus is not a risk factor for HIV infection" (Perez-Stable, 1991, p. 563).

Naturally this approach takes a tremendous toll on individual freedom. The Cubans claim that their program is a humane alternative for HIV-positive persons. Segregating patients, they claim, allows them the opportunity to provide appropri-ate medication, nutrition, and amenities of life that otherwise may be rationed or scarce. Yet others tell a different story. Carlos Otero, for example, is a 17-year-old gay male who has been kept in the Cos Cocos facility outside of Havana since his early teens. Taken from school, virtually imprisoned with hustlers and junkies, he has had no opportunity to continue his education. His own description of life in the facility is like a tale from Charles Dickens. Since his early teens he has witnessed beatings by homophobic guards, suicides and suicide attempts by fellow inmates, and surroundings equivalent to a dismal prison (Bull & Morales, 1995).

Beyond the obvious costs to individual freedom, the long-term success of the policies is questionable. Cuba's quarantine is far from complete. Those infect-ed are allowed occasional, accompanied home visits that can provide at least a small opportunity for the disease to spread. In addition, economically strapped Cuba is actively courting tourism. Tourists will not be tested, thus providing another opportunity for the disease to be spread. Given the possibility of new sources of infection, even mandatory testing would have to be repeated at regular intervals to be fully effective. In fact, the present de-emphasis on the threat of AIDS may even encourage complacency to it.

Responses In the United States

In much of the world, and in the United States, there has been a comparative lack of discrimination and restrictions that were typical in prior encounters with dreaded diseases. In some ways, that may seem surprising. Certainly there were reasons that such restrictions might be expected. First, AIDS was and is a terrifying disease that generated great panics initially. It is a chronic, terminal illness that is debilitating, disfiguring, and communicable. It has all the elements of other diseases that created consternation and consequent restrictions.

Second, the first victims of AIDS were heavily drawn from members of persecuted minorities, engaged in what many considered immoral, and in some areas illegal, behaviors. Gay men, for example, had long experienced both homophobia and varied forms of discrimination. In some states sodomy laws still exist, prohibiting, even in private homes, homosexual acts. Given the facts that homosexuality generated strong antipathy on the part of many in the population and that AIDS was initially perceived in the United States and elsewhere in the West as a gay disease, further restrictions against homosexual behavior would not be unexpected. Some calls for such restrictions are evident. Some have used the AIDS epidemic to decry homosexuality:

> Nearly 75% of those who get the disease are homosexual. And the record is clear the others are indirectly related to homosexuals. . . . Those who are responsible for this epidemic are men and women who are continuing to engage with a wide variety of partners in sexual acts that have been defined as deviant and sinful by the Judeo-Christian community for over 2000 years now. (Fitzpatrick, 1988, p. 34)

There have been calls and attempts for restrictions similar to those of Cuba. For example, Lyndon LaRouche's supporters have called for mass testing and quarantine. Founding a group called PANIC (Prevent Aids Now Initiative Committee) they forced a referendum vaguely mandating restrictive measures on AIDS victims to be placed on the California ballots. Interestingly, more than 70% of 7 million voters opposed the referendum (Bayer, 1989).

Intravenous drug users were even more vulnerable. IV drug use is clearly illegal, considered immoral and self-destructive, and associated with crime. IV drug users were drawn disproportionately from lower income persons of color. Unlike gays, they were unorganized and virtually powerless.

There is evidence of some public support for discriminatory and/or compulsory measures that would be directed against gays. In one study, persons were asked to evaluate a vignette where a company's management forced testing for HIV. They were much more likely to approve compulsory testing for those identified as gay than they were to approve a general policy on compulsory testing (Schwalbe & Staples, 1992). Given this vulnerability, the fact that significant restrictions and discrimination did not occur was remarkable and probably due to four main reasons. First, unlike other minorities, both IV drug users and gays are connected to others, families and friends, who do not necessarily share these behaviors. This can provide a larger, protective umbrella because actions against these groups may have wider, or perhaps more marginal, impact.

Second, the particular characteristics of HIV/AIDS in and of themselves inhibit restrictive behaviors. In its early phases, HIV is asymptomatic. Nor are gay men or IV drug users openly identifiable. Hence, those infected or perceived at risk lack a public visibility that would allow easy identification and subsequent discrimination. Or perhaps the fact that these populations are more marginalized has lessened the public perception of potential threat. In addition, HIV is not transmitted through casual contact and has a comparatively low rate of infectivity. These factors undermine any rationale for restrictive policies because there is a limited public risk. For the most part, one has to voluntarily engage in behaviors to place oneself at risk for transmission.

Third, one clear lesson of the past is that restrictive policies and compulsory health measures are not generally effective in controlling disease. For example, compulsory Wassermann tests for those about to marry did little to dent the rate of syphilis. These policies are even less likely to work in controlling sexual behavior, which is drive-based, and pleasurable or addictive behaviors. Punitive approaches tend to drive such behaviors underground, inhibiting detection, prevention, and treatment. Thus, medical opinion has begun to believe that if individual rights are respected, people will be more inclined to utilize health organizations, facilitating more effective response to the disease.

Finally, and perhaps most importantly, is the entire restructuring of our understanding of rights that emerged from the civil rights struggle. That struggle, begun to ensure equal rights for African Americans, spawned a greater sensitivity to the rights of all, including women, the ill, and the disabled. As a result, there is both a sensitivity to rights and a protective structure of antidiscrimination legislation in the United States at local, state, and federal levels that has served to frame and protect the rights of persons infected with HIV/AIDS. Stoddard and Reiman (1991) see those laws as dramatically changing the ways the United States responds to public health threats such as the HIV/AIDS epidemic.

This does not imply that the AIDS epidemic has not generated strong and contentious debates. Almost from the very beginnings of the epidemic there were intense debates over preventive strategies, civil rights, access to health care, and confidentiality.

The Bathhouse Debate

Perhaps one of the earliest debates and one that would presage forthcoming arguments in preventive strategies was whether bathhouses should be closed. The gay bathhouse was, in many ways, an institution unique to the gay community. Although heterosexual, even bisexual, sex clubs existed, they never had the prominence and participation that the bathhouse had within the gay community. In many communities, the bathhouse was more than an opportunity for sexual liaisons—it was a symbol and community center.

In the post-Stonewall years, the U.S. gay community underwent, as Shilts (1987) described it, a sexual adolescence. After a time of sexual repression, sexual expression and experimentation were now, at least in the major cities, quite open. The bathhouses became a symbol of this sexual freedom as well as a center for gay men to meet. The bathhouses themselves even had their own distinct motifs, select clientele, entertainment, and reputation. Within the bathhouse, patrons could engage in anonymous sex in a variety of ways as well as meet other gay men. It was often one of the first places gay tourists visited.

Yet early in the epidemic, even before transmission of HIV was clearly understood, the bathhouses were identified as likely conduits of disease. Because the more sexually active one was, the greater chance one had of contracting HIV, the earliest victims of AIDS tended to be those who had frequented the bathhouses. Bathhouse patrons too seemed to have higher rates of other sexually transmitted diseases. Shilts (1987) reported that as early as 1982, one physician, Dr. Dan William, approached the owner of New York's largest bathhouse, suggesting that St. Marks should pioneer and educate gay men to a new version of safe gay sexuality that would discourage the anonymous sex and sexual orgies and emphasize video eroticism and mutual masturbation. The request was cavalierly dismissed. There is a certain irony in this, because later when the demands for the closing of bathhouses intensified it was precisely this role that bathhouse owners suggested bathhouses could perform.

Between 1983 and 1985, the debate over bathhouses intensified in the United States. While most of the debate was within the gay community, occasional statements were made by media editorials, politicians, and public health officials and physicians. The argument against the bathhouses was strong. The very existence of the bathhouse, and the sexual opportunities it presented, amplified the choice of exposure and spread of HIV. Shilts (1987) considered it the "single largest element" in the spread of AIDS within the gay community.

But the bathhouse had its supporters. To some, the maintenance of the bathhouses provided a sense of normalcy, a reassurance that the epidemic was not so fearsome, and that moderate changes in sexual behaviors such as limiting partners would minimize the risk of HIV. Some went so far as to minimize the threat of AIDS, claiming that sexual transmission was not proven and gay men were much more likely to die of other causes. To some, too, the bathhouses were a civil liberties issue. Even if they choose not to attend, they reasoned, others should maintain the right to make that choice themselves. There was also the issue of community control. If the gay community acquiesced to the closing of the bathhouse, might not other restrictions follow? Would this not lead to significant curtailments of the rights gays now enjoyed? Then, too, it was argued that bathhouses could have a role in promoting safe sex. Closing the bathhouses, proponents reasoned, would only force sex underground. These arguments were buttressed by the political and economic clout of the bathhouse owners. Many were active members of the gay community, involved in political and charitable organizations and substantial advertisers in gay newspapers. As in past dreaded diseases, this political and economic power, as well as a desire to maintain a sense of community normalcy, proved a significant force for delay.

In gay communities in many major cities, the debate over closing bathhouses intensified into an ugly brawl that fractured political unity. But by late 1984, the debate was largely over. The fear of AIDS and restrictions of sexual activity within bathhouses limited clientele. To politicians, closing the bathhouses had become a way to show resolve in combating the epidemic. In most cities, often with little of the feared protests, the bathhouses closed. Yet this debate clearly showed the complex interplay of forces that continue to make decisions in AIDS prevention contentious and difficult.

AIDS Education

Whereas the debates over the closing of the bathhouses were fought primarily within the gay community, the debates over education became a national debate. In a sense, the earliest debates were between the gay community and some public and religious figures. These debates would foretell the themes that would emerge in broader debates about the role of education in preventing AIDS.

From the beginning, education was seen as having a significant role in prevention. In theory, AIDS, like any sexually transmitted disease, is entirely preventable. If the transmission of the disease to new partners was prevented, the chain of infection would die as its hosts died. Historically, that has yet to happen even in comparatively easily treated diseases such as syphilis. Nonetheless, while it might be unrealistic to assume that education could prevent the disease, it could certainly limit its spread.

From the onset, many gay advocacy organizations such as the New York Gay Men's Health Crisis (GMHC) attempted to educate their own communities. Although some of the initial advice to limit sexual partners and drug use was too conservative, these groups did play a crucial role in educating the gay community. Some of the educational materials they developed were quite explicit. They advocated the use of condoms and emphasized, often with graphic illustrations and full descriptions, safe sexual acts that could substitute for acts that placed participants at risk such as anal intercourse or fellatio. Because some of the materials were supported by public funds, these efforts raised the ire of conservative politicians such as Senator Jesse Helms (R–N.C.) and varied religious leaders.

These debates were a brushfire compared to the controversies that would arise over education in public elementary and secondary schools. Again, given the fact that adolescence is a time of sexual experimentation and experimentation in drug use, there was early concern that children and adolescents needed to be taught about ways to prevent AIDS. This was heightened by the fact that almost a fifth of persons with AIDS are young adults in their 20s, making it likely they were infected as teens. Furthermore, studies of adolescent sexuality show sexual networks of teenagers to be as large as gay networks were in the 1970s (Fulton, 1990). Gay male adolescents and teenage drug users may share special risks.

Given these facts, there has been comparatively little controversy about whether to teach children and adolescents about AIDS. The controversy is over what and how to teach about AIDS. Should adolescents be taught about sexual acts that are of comparatively little risk or should abstinence be advocated? Should they be taught about condoms or have access to them in schools? What should they be taught about homosexuality? Should it be presented as an alternative lifestyle, a moral or psychological failure, or an invitation to disease? Use of illegal drugs presents even more problems. Should adolescents be taught strategies for safer drug use? Should schools distribute clean needles? Finally, how explicit should the language of instruction be? Should sexual acts be described in clinical terms that might be dimly understood or in explicit language of the street?

These questions have generated significant debate on both national and local levels. For example, on a national level, the U.S. Senate recently passed legislation prohibiting the use of federal funds for materials that condone homosexuality. In New York City, the reluctance of the school board to reappoint their chancellor was fed in large part by his advocacy of a "Rainbow Curriculum" that presented homosexuality as an alternative lifestyle as well as his efforts to distribute condoms to high school students. These actions placed him at loggerheads with the politically powerful Roman Catholic hierarchy and engendered strong opposition from more conservative community boards and, ultimately, the city board of education.

Controversies over appropriate education are likely to continue and even intensify as members of movements identified with the religious right seek election to school boards. The content, policies, and presentation of AIDS education are likely to be the spearhead of educational debates.

Drug Prevention and AIDS

Proposals involving preventive efforts to IV drug users have generated even more controversy, because these populations are highly marginal and IV drug use is illegal. Yet the control of the AIDS epidemic in the United States will be achieved only if preventive actions prevail with this population. As Watkins (1988) reminded:

> The future course of the HIV epidemic depends greatly on the effectiveness of our nation's ability to address IV drug abuse. IV drug abusers constitute 25% of all the United States cases. They are a substantial vector for HIV infection, spreading it through the sharing of needles and drug paraphernalia and through sexual contact, as well as perinatally to their children. (p. 849)

Watkins's statement has become prophetic. As the incidence of new cases of HIV among male homosexuals has slowed, it has risen among IV drug users. This risk may even increase as patterns of drug use change. For example, many cocaine users are now injecting the drug. IV drug users may engage in prostitution, both homosexual and heterosexual, to support their habits. And IV drug use represents a significant vector into infecting the adolescent population. Needles, too, may be used by others to inject vitamins, steroids, or medication.

Yet preventive efforts are complicated for a number of reasons. First, the culture of drug users needs to be considered. In a community defined primarily by an addictive need and pervasive poverty, sharing needles is a mark of solidarity because access to syringes may be limited. And, as mentioned earlier, it also provides the secondary user with a "wash," that is, a temporary high derived from the residue of the drug mixed with water. Second, because IV drug use disproportionately affects the Black and Hispanic communities, preventive measures must be culturally sensitive. Third, preventive materials may have to creatively confront constraints of class and culture that may eschew birth control such as condom use, abortion, or even the woman's role in negotiating over sexual acts. For example, in some cultures, it may be considered inappropriate for a woman to possess condoms or suggest a male partner use them. Fourth, there is a barrier of distrust. As Des Jarlais and Stephenson's (1991) research indicates, many persons of color distrust the Public Health Service. These people rejected syringe programs because they thought the government was using needles to spread the HIV virus and kill an unwanted population. Many were well aware of the Public Health Service's role in the Tuskegee study of syphilis.

But one of the biggest constraints is the illegality of IV drug use. Many IV drug users were reluctant to identify themselves to a government agency. This was one factor that limited the effectiveness of attempted syringe exchange programs. For example, New York City's needle exchange program is a good illustration of the difficulties that these programs face.[1] In January of 1988, Dr. Stephen Joseph, New York City Commissioner of Health, was granted permission to conduct a clinical experiment assessing the effectiveness of needle exchange programs for IV drug users. Beyond the distrust and reluctance of IV drug users, the program generated other opposition. Police officials called it "unthinkable." Minority leaders considered it genocide, and a variety of public figures charged it condoned drug use. The program was abandoned 2 years later. Educational efforts at informing IV drug users face similar problems. Many experts suggest explicit materials detailing ways to sterilize needles. There is also a suggestion that materials produced should not condemn drug use but simply focus on behaviors that place one at risk to HIV infections. Others denounce such material as exacerbating drug use and therefore contributing to the epidemic.

Preventive strategies have shown some effectiveness. There is evidence[2] that IV drug users are changing practices toward sharing needles. Yet this too is

[1]See Anderson (1991) for a detailed case study.
[2]See, for example, Des Jarlais and Friedman (1988), Des Jarlais et al. (1988), and Schneider (1988).

affected by the availability of treatment. And if treatment is not readily available, responses to the crisis can be complex. Schneider (1988), for example, reported that IV drug users who tested negative had intense motivation for treatment. Once they tested positive, though, that motivation ceased and many returned to drug use.

Regulation of Sexual Behavior

These debates are prevalent in controversies over other issues. For example, some have called for the intensive persecution of prostitution while others have called for legalization of prostitution. Both sides have claimed that such strategies could reduce the spread of AIDS. Similarly, some have called for increased restrictions on pornography as encouraging unsafe sex. Others have seen it as a possible outlet, deferring sexual acts or providing opportunities to educate or model safe sex strategies.

A similar debate has intensified over the advisability of sodomy laws, still existing in many states and areas, that prohibit homosexual acts. Some have criticized these laws, recently upheld in a divided decision of the U.S. Supreme Court, as inhibiting AIDS education and prevention and discouraging gay men from seeking medical advice. Others have claimed that these laws should be vigorously enforced to prevent AIDS. AIDS has also entered the debate on single-sex marriages. Some have claimed that the legalization of single-sex marriages or the recognition of domestic partnerships can provide a stability and maturity to gay relationships that would inhibit promiscuity. Again, others vehemently oppose anything that would legitimize gay relationships as conducive to the spread of HIV.

Throughout these debates runs a common thread similar to that seen in the debates over syphilis prevention. The most common modes of infection for HIV are activities that are generally illegal such as IV drug use and, in some areas, homosexual acts. Even when these activities are legal, they are considered by some segments of the population to be immoral. Thus, preventive strategies are laced in a paradox. If these strategies explicitly address the behaviors and cultures in a nonjudgmental manner, they are perceived as condoning the behaviors. But if they are moralistic, their effectiveness is likely to be compromised.

The debates that have developed over HIV have paralleled the debates on other dreaded diseases as well. Yet the results, at least in most areas of the world, have been comparatively different. In many past dreaded diseases, restrictions discriminating against the person with the disease were generally instituted. Early in the HIV epidemic, there were many examples of similar restrictions. Schools refused to admit students known to have AIDS. Some airlines declined to serve persons with AIDS. Some funeral directors refused to bury them.

For the most part, however, AIDS victims have been spared the discrimination faced by victims of past dreaded diseases. As mentioned earlier, this has been the result of many factors, including most importantly almost a half century of laws and statutes prohibiting discrimination and a pervasive feeling within the medical community that the more individual liberties are protected, the more likely persons with disease will cooperate with public health.

Mandatory Testing and Contact Tracing

Yet there are still ongoing debates about whether there ought to be mandatory testing for AIDS, either generally or for specific populations, and then whether there should be laws limiting the rights of persons with AIDS.

In a sense that debate began even before a test was available. The debate over screening blood donors began early in the epidemic once blood was suspected of harboring the disease. As early as 1983, Jones Curran, director of the Centers for Disease Control, suggested a highly restrictive donor policy that would include both screening and the maintenance of a registry of those whose blood was deferred. This policy was rejected as violating privacy and being discriminatory. This debate would be a preview of other debates that would distinguish between the rights of the infected individual and others potentially at risk.

In the United States, on a national level, the government does HIV testing for all new armed service recruits and ROTC candidates. Those who test positive are not admitted into the services. There is no requirement, though, that existing personnel who test positive be discharged from the service.

Other than that, the situation varies on a state-by-state, case-by-case basis. Some states, for example, do test applicants for marriage licenses for HIV. This seems of limited value because it is highly cost inefficient and the state's basis for denying a license based on HIV status seems highly dubious.

Some states do require testing of expectant mothers and/or newborns. The rationale here is that early detection of possible HIV infection in babies can enhance early treatment and survival of these infants. However, even this has generated considerable controversy. In New York State, for example, Assembly-woman Nettie Mayersohn proposed a bill in 1994 that would inform mothers of their child's HIV status. In New York such testing is routine but used only for statistical purposes.

Mayersohn and her supporters felt that informing the mother of the child's HIV status can dramatically improve the quality of the child's life by providing early treatment. Mayersohn was opposed by a coalition of gay activists and other supporters who affirmed that mothers should not be tested without informed consent. For if the child is HIV-positive, the mother's own status is HIV-positive. As with other debates, this debate turned bitter, splitting caregivers and civil libertarians. To many AIDS activists, any breach of confidentiality or mandatory testing can create opportunities for other similar requirements. To opponents, the "iron wall of confidentiality" has to be breached to save lives in a public health threat. The final bill passed mandated counseling that would require the mother to make a choice on testing; it would not require testing.

Other states do require testing in situations of sexual crimes. Nevada requires periodic testing of licensed prostitutes. No states yet mandate the testing of health care workers, though some have called for it as well as the testing of a wide variety of professions such as teachers or those involved in the preparation of food.

As the furor in New York over the Mayersohn bill indicated, the debate over mandatory testing is complex. Even beyond the principle of informed consent and confidentiality, there are two other critical issues. First, there is the question of what one would do with results. For example, in the case of blood donor testing, the value is evident. Blood found to be infected would simply not be transfused to others. But in other cases the value is unclear. If there is prenatal testing of expectant mothers, what would occur if they tested positive? Would treatment be mandated? If health care workers tested positively, would colleagues or patients be informed? Would they be restricted in practice? If couples are tested premaritally, would a partner be informed that the other tested positively? Could marriage be denied? Clearly, some of these questions are, or have been, debated. But, for the most part, societal traditions in the United States and in most Western-oriented democracies would inhibit such restrictions.

This leads to the second consideration. Any value of testing would accrue only with the participation of parties involved. The mother would need to decide to undergo treatment. The health care worker would have to evaluate the ways that his or her HIV status affects the practice of the profession. Mandating testing then seems to set a coercive relationship that is not conducive to cooperation.

But the argument over confidentiality has other ramifications as well. As the debate on postnatal testing indicated, it folds into an argument over duty to warn. The duty to warn uneasily coexists with the duty to maintain confidentiality. Present practice tends to allow physicians to breach the latter when it is clear that a given individual is at risk and the patient or client, despite counseling, has no intention to warn. Thus a physician would be within rights to inform a partner or spouse of his or her partner's HIV status.

Ironically, though, it is in the situation where an infected person is sexually promiscuous or engages in risky IV drug use that the law is, at present, most powerless. The illegality of drugs gives the law in the United States some leeway in isolating an indiscriminate HIV-positive IV drug user. But such a person would be difficult to control under today's legal principles and understanding of rights. This is considerably different from past epidemics. Some states do require contact tracing but this is generally seen to be expensive, especially in areas of high prevalence. It is also not likely to be effective. Given the stigma, and possible illegality, of drug use and homosexuality, persons may be reluctant (or even unable) to name their contacts. Beyond the civil liberties dimension, it would certainly seem to discourage testing and be of limited effectiveness. Some states have also considered isolation and have criminalized sexual acts between HIV-positive and other persons. Again, all of these actions seem to be of limited effectiveness, discourage testing, and are difficult to administer in practice.

Other Issues

AIDS has emerged in other debates as well. President Bill Clinton's promise to end restrictions on entry to the United States of persons who were HIV-positive was threatened by the U.S. Senate. The argument of Clinton's supporters was that these restrictions were difficult to enforce because they required voluntary compliance and that generated controversy abroad. This was evident when AIDS activists were denied entry to the United States to attend an international conference on AIDS. Opponents argued that the ban facilitated prevention and protected U.S. health care from assuming the cost of treating HIV-positive immigrants.

AIDS has entered the debate on the future of health care in the United States as well. The AIDS crisis has amplified many of the related problems evident in the U.S. health care system, especially those of cost, equality of access, and universal coverage. Many persons who are HIV-positive have always lived at the margins. They have neither insurance nor assets. Those who do have jobs may find that they have no insurance if they leave or change positions. And employers may find the cost of maintaining insurance prohibitive if they have or place themselves at risk for having HIV-positive employees. Given the difficulty of insurance, who will bear the cost of the crisis, a cost estimated to be $70,000 per patient? In addition, because some HIV-positive persons have insurance and assets, while others do not, a two-tiered system of care could develop.

There have been other debates as well. For example, AIDS activists success-fully challenged the medical community's stance on testing new drugs. The Food and Drug Administration (FDA) historically has moved very slowly and deliber-ately in approving new drugs. Generally this has involved a four-step process that includes preclinical testing with animals, an investigational new drug applica-tion with the FDA, a multiphased human testing process, and a final approval from the FDA. This complete process normally takes years—years that HIV-positive persons may not have. Thus AIDS advocacy groups lobbied for "parallel testing" that would allow new drugs in clinical trials to be available to phy-sicians. In a sense this is consistent with the general direction of other debates. The rights of an individual to take risks gain precedence over a more paternalistic concern of the government to protect persons from unproven drugs.

The debates that have been aroused by the AIDS epidemic are reflective of the arguments evident in previous encounters with dreaded diseases. In each case, the underlying conflict is about how the rights of individuals are balanced against those of the society. What is different about the AIDS epidemic compared to prior epidemics and perceived public health threats is that, in this case, the rights of the individual have been considered paramount. This has been supported by a structure of antidiscriminatory legislation bolstered by two perceptions. The first is that past epidemics have taught that mandatory measures are limited in their effectiveness to stem diseases, especially sexually transmitted diseases. The sec-ond is that once these rights are eroded, society will embark on a slippery slope where the rights of already marginalized groups will be continually threatened.

The Religious Dimension

As with other dreaded diseases, the debates aroused by the HIV/AIDS epi-demic have exposed fault lines within the society as well. In past years, dreaded diseases were often given technological meanings. For example, the varied occur-rences of plague were often pondered for the theological judgment they offered. Cholera and other diseases were also considered by some to be theological judg-ments.

The HIV/AIDS epidemic has come at a more secular time. However, theologians have still found religious explanations of the disease. In effect, the response to the epidemic has illustrated the theological divisions in the contemporary faiths. Kowalewski (1990), for example, has identified three basic religious constructions to the AIDS crisis that basically correspond to the denomination position with the fundamentalist/liberal divide. The more fundamentalist Christian churches and strict Orthodox Jewish sects have seen AIDS as a divine punishment, a chastisement from God for violating scriptural prohibitions against sexual promiscuity, drug abuse, and most particularly, homosexuality. Persons with the disease are seen as touched by divine judgment. Unless they repent of the evil that brought the disease upon them, not only will they suffer in this world, but in the afterlife as well. The language of these groups clearly distinguishes between those perceived as deserving of the disease and those deemed "innocent victims." These "innocent victims" are a judgment against a society far too permissive in allowing such sin.

Members of many traditionalist sects, such as Roman Catholics, the more conservative (but not fundamentalist) Protestant groups, and some conservative Jews, have taken a more middle position. Most of these groups have historically condemned homosexuality as a sin. Yet they would also affirm that individual diseases or those who receive them cannot be seen as personal reflections of God's anger. Sexually transmitted diseases such as AIDS are not necessarily God's judgments but they are examples of what humans bring upon themselves when God's natural laws are trampled. Nonetheless, persons with AIDS should be treated with compassion. Even if one condemns homosexuality as a sin, one still loves the sinner.

The more liberal branches of Christianity and Judaism reject the concept of AIDS as a result of moral failure. These groups have long tended to accept homosexuality as part of the normal range of human sexual expression. Although promiscuity and drug abuse should be avoided, these are often viewed more as social problems than individual failures. If AIDS is a judgment, many of these groups believe it is more a judgment against organized religion for its failure to respond to the disease quickly and compassionately.

Political Debate

The debate over the meaning and response to the HIV/AIDS epidemic is not limited to religion. It has become a major political issue as well, polarized by liberals and conservatives. But interestingly, in many ways it has skewed the ways conservatives and liberals have traditionally viewed governmental roles. In one sense, though, the previous statement is a bit simplistic. The conservative and liberal traditions, at least in U.S. politics, have often reflected broad movements of thought containing many disparate groups and philosophies. For example, the conservative movement today includes essentially those interested in maintaining the status quo, moral conservatives unhappy with contemporary social trends, libertarians, and those actively seeking to find answers to social problems in the voluntary sector. Strains within liberalism are equally distinct and diverse. Characterizing a single liberal or conservative position on the response to HIV/AIDS runs the risk of oversimplifying ideological responses.

That being said, if a conservative position does exist on HIV/AIDS, it is in many ways a departure from more historic conservative positions. Generally, the conservative position has been to minimize the governmental role. In some ways, that has been the response to the HIV crisis. Often conservative politicians have been less sympathetic to increasing government spending for AIDS research and prevention. Many conservative publications such as *National Review* have heralded Michael Fumento's 1990 book, *The Myth of Heterosexual AIDS*. Fumento's thesis is that AIDS represents a minimal risk to heterosexuals. He scorns liberals for trying to "democraticize" the risk and for failing to recognize that gay practices and promiscuity are generally responsible for spreading the disease. To Fumento, the gay lobby, aided by alliance with other liberal groups, has overstated the risk to increase funding. To many conservatives, then, AIDS is adequately funded and any preventive materials should emphasize abstinence from premarital or homosexual sexual behaviors or drug use. In fact, Senator Jesse Helms routinely offers amendments to the fiscal appropriations bill prohibiting funds for any activities that "promote or encourage, directly or indirectly, homosexual, sexual activities." Somewhat ironically, such bills insert a federal role into local discussion on educational curricula or prevention materials.

This departure from traditional conservatism is also seen in other areas. Senator Helms, whom the *Congressional Quarterly* characterizes as leading a congressional faction on AIDS, has also called for mandatory, routine testing; mandatory reporting and monitoring of all HIV-positive persons; criminalization of sexual acts of HIV-infected persons; exclusion of HIV-positive immigrants to the United States; and restrictions on the employment of HIV-infected persons in fields such as health care or education. All of these actions would increase the governmental involvement in health.

The HIV crisis has often led conservatives to vigorously attack the concept of gay rights. In many cases, they have backed state and local initiatives on restricting gay rights. In other cases, they have energetically opposed attempts to repeal sodomy laws. In a 1994 column in the *New York Times*, David Boaz characterized fellow conservatives as obsessed with the issue of homosexuality. He noted that in the past 3 years, the *National Review* had run 32 articles on homosexuality, compared with only 9 on other "family issues" such as parenting, teen pregnancy, and divorce.

Liberals have generally called for increased funding for AIDS research, education, and prevention. Beyond that, liberals, led in the United States by Senator Ted Kennedy (D–Mass.) and Representative Henry Waxman (D–Calif.), have often emphasized both antidiscriminatory legislation prohibiting discrimination against persons who are HIV-positive and inexpensive and confidential testing. The latter emphasis against doing anything to breach the confidentiality of test results has placed liberals in the strange role of limiting the role of governmental public health in the AIDS crisis. For example, in the 1993–1994 session of the New York State legislature, liberals strongly opposed bills allowing victims to know the HIV status of sex offenders, to mandate informing the spouse of persons infected with HIV, or to inform mothers of the HIV status of their child. Most too would oppose doing anything to restrict the reproductive rights of women who are HIV-infected. This is an issue that many conservatives have tended to avoid as well because it would conflict with general positions on birth control and abortion.

Other liberal leaders have called for aggressive prevention efforts including the distribution of clean needles and condoms. Still others have opposed restrictions on the entry of HIV-infected persons to the United States. Some have called for domestic partner legislation that would acknowledge homosexual unions. Others have asked for the decriminalization or legalization of drugs. These latter voices have to be muted because these positions are perceived as politically unpalatable, at least in many areas of the United States. For example, Helms's amendment prohibiting funds that endorse homosexuality passed by a 94 to 2 vote.

Yet these efforts belie a paradox. While there have been efforts to restrict reports, in many ways the AIDS crisis has legitimated the gay community. Gay organizations have become politically astute, using courts and political clout to protect rights. Films and plays have presented compassionate portrayals of gay persons and relationships, and contact between gay organizations and health agencies have in many cities become routine (Altman, 1988). The rising proportion of infected IV drug users has not yet received similar legitimacy.

CONCLUSION

The dangers of the politicization of AIDS have been shown. AIDS has been a comparatively easy issue to politicize. It allows political attacks in the name of public health on generally despised minorities such as gay men or drug users. Such attacks can place opponents in a political dilemma, forcing them to take positions that are either against their instincts or politically dangerous. The result of this politicization is twofold. It polarizes the political debate, creating suspicion and hostility. And it inhibits a thoughtful response to an emerging crisis. The demands of public health become caught in, and subordinate to, an elaborate political game.

Chapter 7

AIDS AS A SOCIAL DISEASE

*Nevertheless, no society could endure the punishment which
the plague had meted out and emerge without serious strains.*
Phillip Ziegler, The Black Death

As one reviews the history of dreaded diseases and the nature of AIDS, two lessons are likely to be drawn. First, dreaded diseases have changed the nature of the societies they afflicted. In some cases, such as the Black Death, their impact is both immeasurable and still debated. In other cases, such as syphilis, the impact seems more subtle but is no less profound.

Second, the AIDS epidemic will profoundly affect the societies it strikes. These effects too are likely to be debated, perhaps far into the future. But these effects are also likely to be significant and long-lasting.

Some sociologists like Fulton (1990) see AIDS as having the potential to be a "species killer," to end the page on the human chapter in the evolutionary process. To Fulton, AIDS may, within a few generations, essentially infect and kill the childbearing generation.

Even if one does not accept Fulton's doomsday scenario, the social impacts of the epidemic are likely to be great. Both the third and developed worlds will experience significant changes. This chapter explores the effects of this epidemic in Africa, which may well model the effects of the disease on the third world, and the United States and the West.

But these scenarios are, as yet, incomplete. The AIDS epidemic will profoundly change the ways humans relate to one another. These social and societal relationships will indeed change. The direction of the change, though, will be determined by the response.

AIDS IN AFRICA: A TALE OF TWO SCENARIOS

Scenarios can be useful ways to explore possible futures. That AIDS will have an impact on the future of Africa is beyond debate. What that future may be is still open. The following scenarios illustrate two alternative futures, or polar examples of the kinds of effects that the HIV/AIDS epidemic may have on the future of Africa.

A Negative Scenario: Africa Desolate Because of AIDS

Colleagues thought he was crazy, but to Dr. Damian Dillon, the AIDS epidemic in Africa represented a virtual calling. Ever since he was a child, he had heard remarkable stories from his mother about Father Damian, a saint who had given his life to live among the lepers. Those stories of self-sacrifice had encouraged his own love of medicine. Zaire seemed the culmination point, the end of a journey he had been destined to take.

Even the airport warnings, listing most of the airports in sub-Sahara Africa as unsafe, did little to deter him. By 2010, Africa had become decimated by AIDS. The scenes depicted in the videos sent by the Centers for Disease Control seemed to him reminiscent of Europe in the grip of the bubonic plague. The social structure, already strained by urbanization, had virtually collapsed. The urban class, separated from their families, had been first to succumb. As urban services deteriorated, there was a return to the villages. But these returnees simply transplanted this new plague with them. Fields lay fallow, conservation efforts ebbed, tourism and trade collapsed, famine reasserted itself. With little employment, armed bands roamed the country. Thousands of desperate AIDS orphans, some of them infected with the virus themselves, were ready recruits. In part, there was self-protection in these bands. Villagers were known to kill whole families of victims of the "wasting disease." Given the chaos and anarchy, foreign aid was reduced to a mere trickle, as donors despaired in the face of multiple problems that seemed impervious to solution.

Damian knew all this as he was strapped into his plane, awaiting take-off. Yet there was challenge to this. One person could make a difference, a far greater difference than one could make in the United States, Damian noted in his diary.

Five days later, when he finally left Lagos, Dr. Dillon was amused by that naivete. Had it only been 5 days? Innumerable obstacles, unconscionable bribes, countless delays—he had expected these. The theft of his luggage and medical supplies and a gunpoint robbery by police in Kinshasa were things he had considered. The mindless, unnecessary raid on his clinic, only hours before he was to start . . . all that battering . . . even that only unnerved him. But it was the consoling offer from a government official, of a night with a prostitute barely in her teens, that convinced him to return to the United States. It was so useless.

AIDS as a Turning Point: A Positive Scenario

Sometimes, Dr. Mufasa pondered, the strangest things became turning points. It had been so for her personally. When she was but a young girl, her father, a trucker on the Trans-Africa Highway, had died of AIDS. Even 40 years later she could remember her mother's wailing. In 2 years, both that mother and a baby brother would succumb to the new disease. Too young to be betrothed, she thought her future seemed short. Then the sisters came—at one point when she was in the orphanage, Mother Theresa herself visited. Dr. Mufasa still remembered the sainted woman holding her hands. "These are warm, beautiful hands," she crooned. "You must be a doctor." Though the sister spoke soothingly, it seemed like a command from God himself. They were hardly beautiful now. Twelve- to fourteen-hour shifts in her hospital, constantly scrubbing, had made them harsh. But they were still the hands of a healer.

But the turning point had been more than personal, it had been a turning point for Africa as well. Long neglected by the rest of the world, the developed world learned that it ignored Africa at its peril. Acknowledging interdependency, nations recognized that by treating persons with AIDS in Africa, they were treating their own. There was reciprocity, too; some folk medicines were proving to be resilient warriors in the battle against this errant virus.

One thing led to another. Prevention programs were coordinated with literacy programs. Medical programs needed local help. A whole cadre of African students, including herself, were trained as physicians. Development aid and peacekeeping forces soon followed.

At times, there were tensions. Western nations, stung by corruption and mismanagement, demanded controls reminiscent of colonial times, generating nationalistic reactions. But this spurred significant political reform movements, led in many cases by junior military officers. They were often inspired by South Africa, which was as aggressive in promoting democracy as it had been in opposing apartheid. In many cases, in fact in most, these coups and popular movements really did reform and democratize. Many countries, such as Zaire and Angola, were truly well endowed. In peace, they prospered. Other countries, troubled by tortuous histories and limited resources, still struggled. It was far from a golden age, thought Dr. Mufasa. But there was hope.

THE EFFECTS OF AIDS IN AFRICA

Which, if either, of these two scenarios will unfold remains open to question. But the encounter with HIV is likely to change the development of sub-Sahara Africa. For AIDS is likely to have long-standing political, economic, and social effects.

The very demography of AIDS in Africa heralds such impacts. To understand the possible effects, it is necessary to review this demography. First, in many areas of Africa, health statistics are notoriously poor. Records are not always kept. Diagnoses, especially in rural areas, may never be made. Many countries may not have set up effective systems for surveillance and reporting. Even when these systems are in place, data, especially from rural areas, may not be forthcoming. In some cases, AIDS cases are simply lost within the last mortality and morbidity rates. And some countries may deliberately underreport to mitigate any negative effects on tourism and economic development.

Second, seroprevalence rates that help estimate the future course of the epidemic are even harder to ascertain. HIV testing is not widespread in Africa. The data that do exist are often drawn from groups such as prostitutes, truck drivers, or blood donors that are not representative of the population. In addition, there is a lack of analogous diseases that could enhance the modeling of seroprevalence rates. Little is known, for example, about the rates of participation in various sexual practices or the progression from infection to disease.

Yet even if data are fragmentary, the resultant morbidity and mortality rates are both staggering and frightening. Barnett and Blaikie (1992) report a Zimbabwe study that suggested that as much as 28.5% of the active workforce in Harare may be HIV-positive. Similar percentages have been found in other nations of the "AIDS Belt" such as Uganda, and Rwanda (Barnett & Blaikie, 1992). As of 1992, close to 9 million adults and children in Africa have been infected with HIV, representing 68% of the total world population so infected. The rate of progression has shown dramatic increases over the past decade. For example, a Kenya study found 3% of men attending sexually transmitted disease clinics in 1981 were HIV-infected. A decade later, that rate had risen to 23% (Mann et al., 1992). Although some rates have seemed to stabilize, now political instability in countries such as Zaire and Rwanda may very well lead to resurgences of infection. Mann et al. (1992) continue to see the disease increasing in Africa in the immediate future and project almost 50% more cases, or close to 13.5 million, currently and anywhere from 21.7 to 33.6 million by 2000. Given the high birth rate of the area, one can then expect population increases to slow or even slightly decline in some countries of sub-Sahara Africa.

These demographic changes are likely to affect social, political, and economic stability. Barnett and Blaikie (1992) offer a scenario describing the economic effects of HIV on an extended family. In this family, some members work in urban areas sending some of their money home. The family runs a small 2-acre farm with crops consisting of staples such as plantain, potatoes, beans, and vegetables, and a cash crop, coffee. The remittances from the sons' working allows the family to hire occasional workers as well as provide for fertilizers, herbicides, and pesticides. As the urban-based children get ill, these remittances cease. The family no longer has help. In addition, because there is no money for fertilizer, pesticides, and herbicides, the family spends more time cultivating a lower yield. As the disease spreads within the family, the eldest child is removed from school to help care for the farm and the infected. Coffee is replaced by cassava because it requires less work. The family's income, though, is reduced. Funeral and medical costs further reduce the family's income. Within a decade, a once stable and comparatively prosperous family is reduced to subsistence levels.

This scenario is played out thousands of times in Africa. A disease that primarily affects persons between 15 and 50 years of age is likely to dramatically affect the supply of labor. In agriculture, this is likely to lead to lower crop yields, particularly in areas already affected by other environmental effects such as low fertility or drought. But these impacts do not end there. Every change has the potential of creating successive changes. As agricultural yields decrease, food security may be threatened. This can generate famine and political instability. Foreign exchange may be lost both as cash crops are reduced and as more money is spent on food and fertilizer. Uncultivated land may fall victim to other pests such as mosquitoes or tsetse flies, increasing the possibility of other diseases.

There may be other effects on economic development. As countries become associated with disease, entry of their nationals to other areas may be discouraged or restricted, limiting remittances sent back to the home country. On the other hand, as labor decreases, particularly in the urban elite, foreign specialists may have to be imported to run the base infrastructure. Tourism and international investment may decline. Multiple losses within the family system may strain extended kin's ability to care for both the young and old, necessitating costs for orphanages and old age homes. In addition, as the epidemic spreads there will be increased needs to expand health services. And health costs are likely to increase, further straining economic development.

The educational system may be affected as well. It is possible that increased funding for health care may come at the expense of education. In any case, the epidemic may affect both the size of the cadre of educators and the availability of students. Educational standards may very well decline with further negative effects on economic development.

There may be indigenous effects as well. Past epidemics have often led to an intensification of religious beliefs and sometimes manifestations of distinct religious movements, such as the Flagellants of the Black Death. The possibility exists that such intensification may occur in Africa. Given that sub-Sahara has large numbers of Christians, Moslems, and animists in some areas, with histories of conflict, the possibility of religiously based conflicts should not be ignored. There are also possibilities of synergistic religions developing that combine religious strains such as Christianity, Islam, and animism or traditional beliefs. Healing cults, based upon charismatic "healers," are quite possible. Especially as the year 2000 approaches, apocalyptic and millenarian cults are likely to arise. Conversely, anomie and despair are also likely to rise.

Sociopolitical effects are likely too. As the disease spreads and economic conditions change, there are likely to be increased population movements. These movements may challenge territorial boundaries and traditional living patterns, increasing intergroup tensions already likely to be strained by declining economic standards. This is particularly dangerous in Africa where colonialism often ignored ethnic boundaries, essentially creating nations from groups that did not share similar cultures and often had antagonistic histories. After the colonial era, these nations did not recognize each other's boundaries and were influenced by the culture of the colonial power. In many of the countries, though, ethnic differences still remain major fault lines.

Previously, epidemics exposed these major fault lines, often leading one group to scapegoat and blame another. The HIV epidemic seems likely to do the same.

Barnett and Blaikie (1992) describe how traditional beliefs and scientific theories are often welded together. For example, in their study, persons acknowledge that AIDS is transmitted by a virus. Yet they may still blame witchcraft for the transmission of the virus in a particular encounter. These explanations provide illustrations of how scientific explanations do not preclude the stigmatization of either individuals or groups. Perhaps the witch burnings reported in South Africa or the genocide evident in Rwanda may be fearful prophecies of the awful possibilities posed by AIDS.

While cultural and religious minorities may lose security and status in the course of the epidemic, so may women. As husbands and sons die, economic security of women is likely to decline. Younger women may become more desirable wives, leaving older women to spend more time in the economically uncertain status of widows. Women's educational gains may be reversed both due to their responsibilities as caregivers and possible strengthenings of traditional beliefs and gender roles.

The AIDS epidemic is likely to challenge African governments. Those perceived as responding effectively to the epidemic may have enhanced legitimacy and even forge new national purpose not seen since the independence struggles. Ironically even new national orphanages have positive possibilities if they can allow the emergence of an educational cadre that transcends ethnic and familial allegiances. On the other hand, the unyielding demands on governmental services can weaken a fragile infrastructure, further eroding authority and control.

The epidemic is likely to increase dependence on foreign donors. The end of the cold war has diminished the strategic importance of Africa, already decreasing incentives for aid. Yet the AIDS epidemic, which has hit Africa harder than other sections of the world, will increase Africa's need. Some have suggested the manifold needs of the continent may create donor fatigue or despair, limiting the ability or desire of other nations to contribute. This may also be affected by conditions in donor nations. Many Western nations are still recovering from economic recessions and are coping with their own HIV epidemic.

But the pressing nature of the needs of Africa, especially as they are acknowledged in the media, is likely to continue to encourage foreign help. In many cases this need is legitimized by international organizations such as the World Health Organization and the United Nations. Then, too, there are continuing ties to former colonial powers and/or cold war sponsors.

It is likely, though, that aid given by international agencies will have stringent controls. The possibility exists then for an indirect "donor colonialism" where the funding agencies exercise significant controls over the ways monies are disbursed. In the stable democracies of sub-Saharan Africa such as Zimbabwe, Namibia, or South Africa, this power is less likely to be exercised. In countries such as Zaire, however, agencies are likely to maintain extensive controls. This role, while likely to create resentment, may also have the paradoxical effect of strengthening democratic movements both by encouraging African democracies and by insisting on democratic changes as conditions for assistance. The effect could be mitigated, however, if donor agencies do not distinguish among govern-ments in setting controls or if the controls are so heavy-handed as to provoke nationalistic backlashes.

Africa, as it enters the next millenium, is a continent poised at the point of transition. Rich in resources, moving beyond the ideological struggles of the past, and beginning to redevelop democratic forms and market economies, Africa may, some believe, experience a great economic spurt. Yet the HIV/AIDS epidemic also will clearly affect its future. The Africa that emerges in the next two decades will be a very different continent due to the HIV/AIDS epidemic. Only the direction of the changes is unknown.

AFRICA: MODEL FOR THE THIRD WORLD?

The course of the disease in Africa may provide an unfortunate model of what may be expected in other developing nations. At present, rates in developing countries vary. Caribbean and Latin American nations have comparatively high rates while the Middle East and Asia presently report comparatively low rates. In Latin America and the Caribbean, heterosexual transmissions have seemed to be the major vehicle of transmission and, as in Africa, gender ratios are nearly equal.

Asia demonstrates the comparative difficulty of slowing the spread of the disease. Despite the fact that the disease did not spread to this area until the early to mid-1980s, preventive efforts already seem too little and too late. For example, studies show dramatic increases of seroprevalence in India of intravenous drug users and sexual workers in India and a growing rate of seroprevalence in Thai-land as well (Mann et al., 1992). As in many parts of the world, the spread of the disease is complex and ever changing. Yet it is also clear that national boundaries will do little to halt the disease.

As in Africa, as AIDS spreads, it is likely to have significant social, political, and economic effects. The economies of these nations vary from comparatively strong to fragile. The economic impacts are, of course, most significant in more fragile, subsistence economies. The impacts on political stability will also vary. In some of these countries, intercommunal strife is high and political/social unity is elusive. In other countries, there is a strong sense of shared history and culture that bolsters unity. Thailand and India provide good illustrations of the potentially differential effects of the HIV epidemic on political and social unity. Both nations seem to be in the early phases of what is likely to be a significant epidemic. In Thailand, though, the sense of social unity is strong. The epidemic is not likely to fracture that unity. In fact, if the monarchy takes a leadership role in preventing AIDS, by abolishing sexual tourism and advocating health services for the HIV-infected, the monarchy may continue to consolidate its prestige and influence. And such nonpolitical roles have, in fact, been traditional roles of the monarchy. Already the army, traditionally a significant player in Thai political and social life, has begun to take a significant role in HIV education and prevention. Such an active role may do much both to stem the rising tide of infection and to buttress the army's critical role.

The HIV/AIDS epidemic, though, may fracture India's fragile unity. Like Thailand, India is likely to be an Asian epicenter of the disease. India is at particular risk for three reasons. First, India does have a population of intravenous drug users. Second, India has a large pool of paid blood donors, many of whom sell blood in less than sterile conditions. Finally, prostitution is not uncommon in India, buttressed by poverty, urbanization, and in some cases, even religious ritual.

India has long struggled with intercommunal strife and separatism. Because plagues often expose fault lines within a society, AIDS may very well be the fuse that ignites India's communal tensions.

In India, the challenge of the emerging epidemic will be to defuse the intercommunal tensions that may grow in the wake of the disease. In fact, should the central government be perceived as ineffectively responding to the epidemic, intensification of separatist movements and intercommunal violence could continue to rise and sunder the state.

AIDS IN THE WEST: TWO AMERICAN SCENARIOS

AIDS will also continue to affect American society. Again, here too, the effects may lead to different alternative futures. The effects are already evident in the gay community. These widespread effects will spread throughout other segments of American society as well. The two following scenarios are incomplete in that they only explore how the HIV/AIDS epidemic may affect American attitudes toward homosexuality. Surely it will affect those. But it will also affect much more, including the very fabric of social relationships.

A Wedding: AIDS as a Force for Tolerance

It was a bittersweet moment for Anthony as he raised a toast celebrating Kevin and Terry's life partnership. He had met Kevin, so many years ago it seemed, as a volunteer in an AIDS program Anthony had joined after his own lover, Jim, had died. Anthony, 20 years older, had become a mentor, almost a father, to the young, idealistic Kevin. It was a wonderful relationship, a great friendship. Sex had never been a part of it. Their relationship was such that sex would seem almost akin to incest.

But Anthony had schooled Kevin in the movement's history—the pre-Stonewall days, the heady days of liberation, and the plague.

He thought about Jim. To Jim, sex was almost—hell, it was—a political statement—an in-your-face, out-of-the-closet statement. It was a celebration of sexuality, of promiscuity in a society that barely tolerated his homosexuality. How many times had Jim mocked Anthony's own sense of monogamy, his conservatism.

It was that caution that saved him from the plague that cut down Jim so early. Jim's last words were meant to be a comforting "for better or worse." It had been what Anthony had wanted, a forever kind of commitment, the kind Kevin and Terrance were promising in front of a judge in a Sutton Avenue townhouse rented for the occasion. It was ironic that it was that very plague that allowed this very public and all too legal ceremony. The AIDS crisis had led first to medical insurance allowing domestic partners to be covered on one another's policies. Then there was a legal procedure to register. Soon it took all the ridiculous trappings of a conventional wedding. But that was too positive. The judge intoned about the need to stabilize relationships, to remain faithful to one another. Anthony's thoughts drifted back from Jim. Terrance and Kevin had found a good way, perhaps the best way, to fight the plagues, or disease, that consumed Jim, and the loneliness that sometimes, often now, engulfed him.

The Sentence: AIDS and Homophobia

Six months probation and a $1,000 fine. It seemed incredible, totally amazing, really, to an old activist like Adam, that he had actually been convicted of a sodomy crime. In 2012! In Las Vegas! His lawyer kept reminding him he was lucky. Had he been HIV-positive, had his partner not known, he could have been imprisoned for life. In some states like Alabama, that was even a capital crime.

Another old movement figure had reminded him it always goes in cycles. Eventually, he counseled, these laws will be overturned or ignored. You can't fight nature.

Adam wasn't so sure anymore. In 1997, a cluster of AIDS cases had been uncovered at Penn State. Sixteen kids, heterosexual, White suburban kids, one only in middle school, had been infected by the disease. A panic ensued.

The AIDS riots took place that summer. Poor Black and Hispanic communities, outraged at the response to the "Penn State 16"—the new funding, new laws—reacted with a burning indignation that their own pain had been so long ignored. To Adam, their indignation matched his own.

They didn't seem to think so, though. It was the gay communities and clubs that the rioters targeted. It was gay men who were grabbed off subways and buses and cars, beaten, killed.

All these events fed in so well to the apocalyptic prophecies of the next millennium. People were scared. AIDS had come home.

He did not believe the new laws—outlawing homosexuality, drug use, pornography, even sexual encounters—would work. You cannot enforce laws like that, he thought, as he accepted the receipt for the fine.

THE EFFECTS OF THE EPIDEMIC
IN THE UNITED STATES

These two scenarios represent possible, even plausible, alternative futures that may result from the HIV epidemic. As in Africa, the potential impacts of the epidemic are difficult to ascertain. Unlike Africa, in the United States and in many sections of the West, AIDS is still a disease on the margins. Despite all the publicity, attention, and fear AIDS generates, it still represents a disease of the Other Americans. It remains a disease associated with gay men or IV drug users. And it is gay men or persons of color whom the disease is seen primarily as affecting. In fact, one of the major factors that will determine the effects this epidemic has will be whether the disease begins to show similar patterns of transmission as found in the third world. If heterosexual transmission, especially involving non–IV drug users, becomes more common and heterosexually active persons, both adults and adolescents, become more generally infected, the course of AIDS in the United States may take a very different turn. This spread is increasingly likely to occur. In analyzing data from the CDC, Kennedy and Fulton (1995) conclude that the HIV epidemic has now reached a "third stage" in the United States. The first two stages represented those in high-risk groups (men engaged in homosexual activity, IV drug users, and blood recipients) and then their sexual partners. The emerging third stage represents a significant expansion of the epidemic as low-risk heterosexuals and sex partners of second stage persons begin to become infected.

Yet even in that circumstance, the turn AIDS will take is still unclear. Even De Tocqueville's classic study, *Democracy in America*, written in 1835, found an America full of internal contradictions. It professed a creed of equality and an ethos of freedom, yet kept persons enslaved. Similar contradictions abound today. Americans pride themselves on being free thinkers, yet Americans are by far more religious than European counterparts. Sexual experimentation has uneasily coexisted with a strong sense of puritanism. Conservative and progressive tendencies and values persist in almost all social classes and groups. The political liberalism of the African American community, forged in the civil rights struggle, can mask the social conservatism of the Black church. Americans may abhor certain behaviors, but they tolerate those behaviors in individuals who remain discreet and inoffensive. They can be simultaneously angry and openly generous. They may despise welfare, resenting those who they feel abuse the system, while at the same time running food and toy drives for these very same persons. In the United States, the 1994 elections exemplified that ambivalence. In many areas, the electorate opposed anti-gay initiatives often in reaction to an intolerance that many found disturbing. But in other areas and in polls, voters have shown a marked reluctance to take actions that would seem to legitimize a homosexual lifestyle. The Clinton presidency's compromise on gays in the military— "don't ask, don't tell"—seems emblematic of a national response to sexuality.

It is these contradictions that make forecasting so difficult. One can never be sure of which currents the epidemic may tap. And past history shows it could tap several simultaneously. During the cholera epidemic in the 1840s, the Irish Catholic immigrants were often blamed for the disease even while their clergy, generally held in suspicion, were commended for their compassion.

The AIDS epidemic is likely to expose fault lines within American society. As discussed in earlier chapters, there are already distinct liberal and conservative positions on AIDS that seem to be reasonably consistent despite the disparate strains of each movement. The epidemic has exposed similar divisions within and between religions, as also discussed. But AIDS is likely to expose other fault lines as well.

Certainly social divisions may be accentuated. Dalton (1989) noted that the African American community harbors deep resentment over AIDS. First, it has fueled suspicion and mistrust of the White community. In some cases, this mistrust has been fueled by perceived attempts to blame Blacks for the disease by focusing on African origins and Haitian roles in transmission. In other cases, there was an underlying suspicion that this virus may in fact have been willfully spread by the government to eliminate perceived undesirables. Even if this was not planned, calls for abortion of HIV-infected children may be seen by some segments of the Black community as a form of genocide (Dalton, 1989). Then, too, Dalton (1989) noted this feeds the resentment of "White neocolonialism," that Whites are both dictating action and absorbing most of the funding. Dalton (1989) also noted that the Black community is defensive over the association of drug abuse that evokes some of the racist images evident in the syphilis epidemic.

But the AIDS epidemic may also expose tensions within the Black community. The African American community has shown remarkable political cohesiveness historically. Both the abolitionist and civil rights struggles defined a common political agenda that transcended other divisions. Yet these divisions may grow as the AIDS epidemic continues. Dalton (1989) suggested that homophobia may be more intense in the Black community because it evokes uncomfortable images, associated with enslavement, of strong women and weak men. In addition, homosexuality may be blamed for a disease that is decimating many minority communities. Homosexual behaviors are also condemned within many conservative religious traditions, whether Christian or Islamic, that find expression within the Black community.

These tensions have already strained relationships with the activist gay community, which is a traditional ally in rights struggles. It may in the future fracture political unity within the Black community, creating conflicts between progressive and conservative political factions.

The gay community in the United States is itself facing similar stresses. On one hand the AIDS crisis has provided a common front. Legislation prohibiting discrimination against persons infected with HIV and protecting confidentiality as well as health policies that provide increased spending and faster testing of drugs are issues that have widespread support. On the other hand, tensions over "outing" or exposing to the larger community homosexuals who have not publicly declared themselves seem to have increased, with some gay activists claiming it is a duty in the midst of an epidemic to affirm one's sexuality because it brings the crisis closer to individuals who may think themselves removed. Shilts (1987) also indicated tensions between those who do not warn of an infection or take appropriate action to prevent infection and other members of the gay community. Shilts (1987) also suggested ongoing conflicts between those who favored a new definition of gay sexuality based on themes of liberation and openness and those who looked toward more traditional views of monogamous couples. All of these tensions have been muted in the quest of beleaguered minority to maintain a united front in the face of a frightening epidemic. But all may become more open and conflictive as the epidemic continues. In fact, some gay groups have already questioned that very basis of unity, asserting that the AIDS crisis has overwhelmed other more contentious issues within the gay community that can no longer be ignored.

General social attitudes toward sexuality in the United States are ambivalent, shaped by both a puritanical Judeo-Christian heritage and social libertarianism. As a result, Americans have tended to have negative attitudes toward homosexuality while at the same time tolerating homosexuals who stayed within whatever discreet boundaries were defined at the time. This is further buttressed by the fact that many Americans are likely to have family members, friends, or coworkers who are openly, or suspected to be, gay.

This is not to say that social tolerance or acceptance of homosexuality is openly embraced. Violence against homosexuals is still reported nationally. In some areas, homosexuality is still against the law. And as Chapter 6 indicated, debates about homosexuality still continue.

The HIV epidemic will affect this tenuous tolerance of homosexuality. Some factors may increase or bolster tolerance. Media images of persons with HIV such as the television movie *An Early Frost* or the award-winning feature film *Philadelphia* underline, in a compassionate way, a common humanity. And as gay individuals suffer through the illness, their families, friends, and communities may be forced to confront homosexuality in a very different way. It may be more difficult to deny another's sexuality.

At the same point, tensions can increase. Calls for increased spending on the disease have already begun to rankle advocates for other illnesses. Increased gay activism has generated reactions. At present, though, the patterns of blame and scapegoating so evident in other epidemics have not occurred. A number of factors account for that. First, Americans, as stated earlier, have always had an ambivalent response to sexuality. Second, U.S. multiculturalism as well as more than 30 years of varied civil rights struggles have produced both an ethos of tolerance and a broad structure of antidiscriminatory legislation. This tolerance then is tenuous but unlikely and it may be dramatically challenged as the epidemic in the United States changes course. Should, for example, HIV begin to be more widely perceived as a disease threatening other groups, such as middle class sexually active adolescents and young adults, that tolerance could be staunchly threatened.

If the disease does continue to spread to other risk groups, it is more likely to occur through IV drug users. The HIV epidemic is likely to create continued pressure to deal effectively with drug use. Because it is difficult to prevent the risk of HIV infection among IV drug users, efforts probably will be aimed at preventing serious drug use. Although such methods may be less than effective, it is also probable that the approach will be punitive, mandating treatment and/or longer prison terms for those involved in selling or using drugs.

In summation, the HIV epidemic will, like most dreaded diseases, expose political, religious, and social fault lines. Even geographic fault lines are likely to be exposed as cities more than suburbs and coastal areas more than middle America cope with the crisis. As long as the HIV epidemic remains marginalized, these effects are likely to be muted. But if the epidemic moves beyond the risk groups, past experience suggests accentuation of conflicts.

The HIV epidemic is also likely to change the face of health care in the United States. Two effects of the epidemic are most immediate. The first is cost. HIV infection is a chronic disease with a complex and heavy treatment regimen. Costs for the disease include not only the costs of treatment but diagnosis of AIDS-related conditions such as dementia. In addition, there are costs for prevention and research. These costs are likely to increase as more persons are diagnosed earlier in the disease, leading to earlier treatment, and persons live longer with the disease. Mann et al. (1992) estimated that approximately $2.3 billion was spent for care of persons with AIDS in 1992. This figure will increase significantly by the end of the decade.

The HIV epidemic will not only contribute to rising health care costs, it also will accentuate the problem of health care access. In 1990–1991, 29% of persons with AIDS were uninsured; another 40% were insured through Medicaid (Mann et al., 1992). It is little wonder that there is continued pressure to radically restructure U.S. health care systems to both control costs and provide universal coverage. This is likely to continue to remain a major political issue.

Other effects of the HIV epidemic on the medical system are also likely. Some infected by HIV are highly sophisticated persons, suspicious of the health care systems. Others may be less sophisticated but equally suspicious. The result is, much as in cancer, an extensive alternative medical network that embraces everything from complementary therapies such as imaging to underground systems for obtaining untested or unapproved drugs to folk healers. To the extent that standard medicine is unable to stem the epidemic, this network will grow. In addition, there may be increased pressures on the Food and Drug Administration to continue to loosen its regulations on the testing and approval of new drugs.

Other significant social changes can be expected. In 1994, untoward comments by the new Republican Speaker of the House of Representatives, Georgia Congressman Newt Gingrich, that there might be a need for orphanages were roundly criticized by child care advocates. The context of the Speaker's comments was that orphanages might provide a way of welfare reform, breaking multigenerational cycles of dependency. Orphanages, though, could also be a result of the AIDS epidemic. In the mid-1800s, the cholera epidemic fostered the development and growth of the orphanage. A century later, other demographic changes such as improved mortality and morbidity, smaller families, and a developing foster care system closed most of these orphanages. Levine and Stein (1994) estimate that by the end of the decade as many as 125,000 U.S. children will be orphaned by AIDS. Many of these children will be older children of color. Some of them will come from families that are highly dysfunctional, the offspring of IV drug users. Foster care systems, especially in large cities, may be unable to meet the demand. It is not unlikely that there will be new orphanages built in the next decade.

Other changes in the United States may be the result of AIDS as well as other factors. Both Cornish (1986) and Johnston and Hopkins (1990) see a new sexual restraint that may very well lower current divorce rates. Johnston and Hopkins also foresee a new pessimism. This is possible in the United States, for not since 1918 has an epidemic primarily killed the young. Thus the idea of continued progress, people living longer and happier lives, may be a casualty of the AIDS epidemic, particularly on the young.

Other effects ripple through the society at large with perhaps little notice. Yet the HIV/AIDS epidemic continues to create and influence new and existent services in so many ways. For example, the gerontological network, consisting of home health care, nursing homes, and other services such as meals on wheels, has expanded its mission to include persons infected with HIV. Whole new industries have developed in response to the epidemic. For example, the viatical industry has emerged in this epidemic. Viatical companies pay a cash value for life insurance policies, providing funds for individuals struggling with illness.

Other effects of the disease are incalculable. Its effects on fashion, theater, and other arts, areas where many homosexuals traditionally found a level of acceptance, are impossible to ascertain. Who can determine the pieces uncompleted, the plays unwritten? These areas especially abhor vacuums. Others will fill these niches. Only in retrospect will one be able to judge in what ways the course of these fields were modified by the disease. How will the deaths of so many creative people in the prime of their lives—Arthur Ashe, Greg Louganis, Michael Bennet, Randy Shilts, to name just a few—affect society? These effects are essentially incalculable.

It is also interesting to speculate on the ways that AIDS will affect the transition into the next millennium. Turns of the centuries have historically been times of torment, anxiety, and millenarian movements. This may very well be the wild card, the discontinuity in forecasting the future of AIDS. A charismatic leader, evoking the spectre of AIDS in the context of the next century, has the potential to shape the response to the disease.

AIDS IN EUROPE

It is beyond the scope of this book to explore the impacts of the disease on the rest of the industrial world. In many ways, many of the effects of the disease in the United States will be echoed throughout the industrialized world. Two implications in Europe are worth noting. Since the 1960s, European nations have done much to erase national borders. One unfortunate result of this has been the movement of intravenous drug users throughout Europe. This mobility has complicated treatment and prevention (Mann et al., 1992). It is possible, although at this point still unlikely, that attempts to control this population may reverse this historic trend.

Another group in Europe that may be affected are immigrants, particularly from the third world. Many European countries, including England, France, and Germany, have had anti-immigration movements of varying size and political importance. The AIDS epidemic may very well accentuate these currents. Immigrants have not been a major contributor to the AIDS epidemic in Europe, but they have been a factor. Many European nations retain strong ties with former colonies in Africa and have significant numbers of migrants from these central African countries (Shannon et al., 1991). In addition, many persons from Africa travel to Europe for medical care. Given the disparity in expenditures and levels of care for HIV infection, this is likely to be more common. There is a strong possibility that the AIDS crisis will lead to increased calls to restrict immigration in Europe.

CONCLUSION

In summary, the HIV/AIDS epidemic provides a case study of the interplay between disease and society. Social changes, in modes of transportation or sexual mores, to name a few, create new opportunities for heretofore unknown diseases to emerge. Once these diseases do come forth, they continue to influence all sorts of secondary societal shifts, revealing the very fragile and tenuous nature of the social order. The society that finally results in the aftermath of this disease is likely to be significantly transformed from the society that existed at its onset.

Thus the HIV epidemic is likely to have many effects, but among the most dangerous, common to past dreaded diseases, is that it can be the "Great Divider," exacerbating existent and dormant tensions. In developing policies to meet the epidemic, it will be critical to maintain and to bolster social unity even in the face of the disease.

Chapter 8

CREATING
A HUMANE FUTURE

To change is the challenge of suffering.
Nathan Kollar, Songs of Suffering

Much of the discussion so far has addressed the HIV/AIDS epidemic from a historical and sociological perspective. The discussion has emphasized that the HIV/AIDS epidemic has arisen from changes in our social organization that have provided opportunities for the virus to spread and become embedded within the population. The book, particularly in the last two chapters, has stressed that this epidemic is likely to dramatically change the societies it affects as did other dreaded diseases in our past.

Yet as Chapter 7 indicated, these changes do not have to be entirely negative. The HIV/AIDS epidemic has the potential for creating considerable social havoc and conflict. It can exacerbate social tensions and pressure medical and caregiving systems. But it can also provide the impetus, as past epidemics did, for innovations in our policies and systems of care. And perhaps it can even challenge us to transcend the divisions and unite in new ways to create a humane future in the face of plague.

This chapter explores the possibilities. Specifically it addresses four issues. First, the ways in which our society can work to prevent HIV infection are addressed. Second, this chapter considers how we may care for those already infected with the virus. A third section discusses the needs of all affected by the virus. HIV will affect many not infected with the virus. The epidemic will leave orphans as well as bereaved family members and caregivers. A final section reviews trends, projections, and recommendations. In assessing these four areas, two concerns are primary. It is important to consider how policies and systems may need to be modified to respond to the epidemic more effectively. Yet it is equally important to consider the qualities and skills that individual caregivers need as they respond to the infected and affected.

AIDS AS AN INTERNATIONAL ISSUE

It is beyond the scope of this book to explore the international actions that will be necessary to respond to this epidemic. Nonetheless, international cooperation will be critical, especially to prevent the HIV/AIDS crisis from becoming a divisive issue between nations and blocks of nations. The recognition that AIDS can have that role is important because past epidemics of dreaded diseases have amply demonstrated the social conflicts that diseases can expose and exacerbate. In addition, there is ample motivation for cooperation because the HIV virus has the capability of eliminating the human race, because it is spread through sexual activity and primarily infects humans in their reproductive years.

Both past experience and contemporary studies have reinforced two lessons. First, compulsory health measures are more often responses to the fears generated by the disease rather than effective strategies for preventing its spread. Second, educational approaches alone will not stem the epidemic.

Mann et al. (1992) emphasize that educational and informational programs have to be specifically targeted and culturally sensitive toward the groups they wish to reach. For example, the term "bodily fluids" used often in U.S. prevention literature avoided offense but at considerable cost to clarity. In addition, information has to be buttressed by appropriate health and social services. It makes little sense to emphasize condom use if condoms are unavailable, too expensive, or culturally foreign. Finally, there must be a supportive social environment that empowers individuals to make appropriate choices rather than try to constrict those choices.

On the international level, a number of actions may be helpful. First, there needs to be a continued concerted, international effort to stem the epidemic. This effort would include facilitating the exchange of information and research and coordinating the testing of potential vaccines. These actions are presently in place and need to be expanded and coordinated.

But other international efforts need to supplement these activities. There needs to be the equivalent of an "AIDS Marshall Plan" for Africa and other sections of the developing world. This plan should strive to assist developing nations in creating a medical and social service infrastructure capable of responding to the HIV epidemic; ensure free and accessible HIV testing; and assist with the research, development, dissemination and evaluation of culturally appropriate educational and informational materials aimed at preventing the spread of HIV.

In addition, international efforts ought to be specifically directed in three other directions. In many developing nations such as Thailand or the Philippines, commercial sex workers have had a role in the spread of the disease. However, sexual tourism is unlikely to lessen without both concerted governmental action and alternative opportunities for economic development.

Second, intravenous drug use is both a worldwide problem and a significant vector in spreading the disease. Again, international efforts will be needed to inhibit the production and distribution of drugs as well as provide alternatives to economic development. The HIV/AIDS epidemic has demonstrated how interconnected our world has now become.

Third, a significant lesson from past epidemics emphasizes that major social changes often disturb the delicate ecological balance between humans and their parasites. The pace of change continues to quicken, suggesting that HIV infection may be the first of many new diseases to trouble humankind. Past evidence of outbreaks of Lassa, Marburg, and Ebola fevers suggest that such diseases are first likely to appear in equatorial climes. The international community would be well served by a number of health stations in remote equatorial zones that could monitor any such diseases and provide an early warning system. Had such a system existed in the 1960s, the history of the HIV epidemic might have been far different.

Beyond these broad strokes, each nation must develop its own policies to prevent the spread of HIV. Such policies will need to be sensitive both to the demographics of the disease and to the social and sexual mores in each particular country.

PREVENTION

Creating the Context for Prevention: Research, Law, and Policy

In the United States, prevention still will remain a critical part of the response to the epidemic. But in order for prevention efforts to be more focused there is a need to increase our knowledge of affected populations. For that reason funding for research about HIV should continue to be a major priority. In recent years there has been some criticism of the level of funding.

It is true that for the number of persons infected with the disease, AIDS research is funded at a comparatively high level. However, evaluating spending on that basis only neglects four facts. First, as an infectious disease, AIDS has the potential to infect significantly more persons than are presently infected. Second, because AIDS presently infects more marginal communities, it has the potential to create increasing alienation and conflict. Third, as a disease of primarily young adults, AIDS has significant economic effects that will increase as the disease spreads. Finally, research on AIDS is likely to have significant secondary and tertiary effects. For example, drugs developed to work against HIV infection may have broad antiviral applications. Vaccines manufactured to prevent AIDS will create new technologies that may assist the development of vaccines for a wide variety of diseases, including more effective vaccines for influenza. And research on AIDS will further probe the nature and role of the immune system, including its part in diseases such as cancer.

In fact, it will be necessary to continue to fund social science research on the disease. For example, considerable research is needed about compulsive and addictive behaviors. In addition, information about the subcultures currently suffering from the disease such as the IV drug culture, the gay culture, and urban Hispanic and African American cultures will not only contribute to broader understanding but will also foster culturally effective preventive efforts.

There are policy issues as well. Testing remains one of the most powerful tools in combating HIV. The more persons who are aware of their HIV status and act accordingly, the more effective prevention and treatment are likely to be. Testing ought, then, to be confidential, easily accessible, and low cost and/or free. This does not mean that testing should not be compulsory in certain contexts. For example, the HIV testing of infants, especially in high-risk communities, can allow early identification and treatment of infected children. At present, requiring HIV tests for other purposes such as marriage licenses or as a condition for immigration does not seem cost effective or necessary. HIV testing presently done by the armed services seems a reasonably effective way to continue to assess the course of the epidemic.

Naturally, HIV testing can be effective only if supportive services are available. For example, counseling, social services, and adequate health care should be accessible. Any pre- or postnatal counseling should provide opportunities for family planning, including information and access to birth control and, if there are subsequent pregnancies, accessible abortions as well as assistance in providing permanency planning for infected mothers. Such planning allows an infected mother to plan for guardianship of her children should she die or become unable to parent.

HIV testing is only likely to occur in a context where individuals feel safe in knowing the results of such a test. Confidentiality should generally be maintained. Laws prohibiting discrimination against HIV-positive persons ought to be reviewed, strengthened if necessary, and vigorously enforced.

There needs to be review of current laws and policies that affect the HIV epidemic. For example, laws against sodomy that prohibit homosexual behavior are generally unenforced and probably unenforceable. Because they may provide a barrier for gay men seeking HIV testing or treatment, they should be revoked. In fact it would make sense to recognize and acknowledge a wide range of domestic unions. This would have two major advantages. First, it would provide additional sanction and support for monogamous relationships. Second, it would strengthen the web of insurance.

Laws against drug use and policies regarding drug use also need consideration. At the very least, methadone treatment has seemed to stem HIV infection. Funds for treating IV drug use should be a major priority. The distribution of sterile needles needs continued evaluation. It may very well be that the HIV crisis will lead to serious national debate about the regulation of illegal drugs. In that debate, decriminalizing drug use and treating it as a medical problem should be considered as a viable option.

The treatment of prostitutes also needs review and debate. The commercial sex industry has been historically resilient to say the least. And it is debatable to what extent in this country commercial sex workers have served as a vector of disease. Nonetheless, data from other countries suggest they can have a significant role in spreading the disease. Legalization and regulation (e.g., mandating condom use) of the commercial sex industry as practiced in some areas of the

United States may have little effect on the large underground of streetwalkers who are most at risk for transmitting AIDS. Nonetheless, there needs to be continued assessment of the role of prostitution in spreading AIDS as well as the effects of strategies such as legalization, education, or vigorous suppression of prostitution to minimize the destructive threat that prostitution poses to the disease.

In addition, laws and policies involving confidentiality need to be reviewed. In general, the principle of confidentiality should be supported. However, no rights are absolute. The most essential mandate to public health is to effectively stem the epidemic and treat those with the disease. In *Tarasoff v. Regents of the University of California*, the courts did determine that counselors have a duty to warn others in danger. There is a legal precedent for health care workers and public health officials to vigorously act when someone who is warned that he or she is HIV-infected fails to inform or warn partners and continues to engage in unsafe behaviors. Ethics committees should be empowered and supported should professionals determine a duty to warn. In the same way, victims of sex crimes should have a right to be informed of the HIV status of a convicted offender. Although this may not demonstrably change the victim's own health practices such as HIV testing, it may alleviate the anxiety produced by uncertainty.

In other cases, the right of other professionals to know a person's HIV status may be supportable if knowledge can help them to assess and avoid risks. For example, principals and school nurses ought to be informed if a student is HIV-positive. However, confidentiality should only be breached in serious and considered circumstances, after efforts are made with the infected individual to inform, and when buttressed by strong laws prohibiting discrimination.

In summary, prevention efforts always take place within a broader context. The context that has historically been most helpful is one that is reasonably noncoercive, offering support and protection to those infected with disease.

Educational Strategies for Prevention

This book has presented two paradoxical principles about the role of education in prevention. First, it is essential. HIV/AIDS is a preventable disease. Helping inform individuals about ways to limit or eliminate behaviors that can expose them to the disease is a moral mandate. On the other hand, the history of sexually transmitted diseases reminds us that educational efforts are unlikely to eradicate the disease given the addictive and compulsive natures of risky behaviors.

Nonetheless, education represents the first line of defense in HIV/AIDS prevention. In the United States there has been considerable debate about what the educational message should be. Yet this debate has generated more controversy than clarity. The prevention of HIV infection is best viewed in the larger context. Sorenson (1991) speaks of lines of defense. For example, the best defense against HIV infection through drug use lies in abstinence. However, if one does use drugs, it will lower the risk if one does not inject drugs intravenously. If one is an IV drug user, a next line of defense is not to share needles, or at least to use clean needles. Similarly, abstinence is the best defense against sexually transmitted HIV infection. However, if abstinence is not used, monogamous relationships, safe sex, and the use of condoms remain subsequent lines of defense. This model reminds one that at each line of defense, the risk of infection can increase. And it reaffirms that the distinction between abstinence versus safe sex/condoms or drug use is not one of opposites. All need to be taught as part of the strategies toward prevention.

Different organizations may have distinct perspectives of where they wish to provide emphasis. For example, drug treatment groups may make the assumption that much of their membership may continue to struggle with drug use. Therefore, strategies of defense other than abstinence may be stressed. Religious organizations may wish to explicitly reinforce their own value systems with their members, especially their young. The messages of abstinence and monogamy are likely to find renewed receptiveness in the age of AIDS.

Schools, though, should provide a comprehensive perspective, allowing their students, at appropriate ages, to use this information as they make their choices on how to best prevent infection. Education about HIV has to become an essential part of health education curricula at all educational levels. This would probably best be done if mandated at the state level.

Although education about HIV/AIDS should be supported at the highest levels of state educational boards, it is critical to establish priorities based upon local needs as well as be sensitive to local mores. For example, communities with high rates of drug use may particularly wish to emphasize strategies designed to prevent the transmission of the disease through intravenous drug use. Communities with high rates of HIV infection may want to place emphasis and spend more time on HIV/AIDS and general preventive strategies. Developing advisory councils consisting of parents, teachers, community members, and even upper level students may be effective ways to engender local support and tailor programs to area needs.

HIV/AIDS education, however modified for given communities, ought to provide information in four major areas. First, it should provide information about

HIV infection, rooting it in the context of communicable diseases. This is critical for a number of reasons. Placing HIV infection in a context of diseases can lessen fears by emphasizing that HIV infection is one of many diseases that can infect humans. An additional point—that HIV is difficult to transmit compared to other diseases—can also lower anxiety.

That information provides a background for a second critical objective in HIV/AIDS education, perhaps its most important objective—to stress that the disease is totally preventable. Children should, at age-appropriate levels, be given both comprehensive information about strategies for prevention as well as skills and practices for a healthy lifestyle. For example, given the levels of sexual activity and drug use in American adolescents, education at this level should empower students to assess strategies of both abstinence and safer sex and/or drug use. In addition, students should be taught strategies of negotiations as well as how to evaluate risk situations. It will help adolescents to identify contexts in which they are likely to engage in risky behaviors. In addition, they may need to learn the social skills for negotiating when placed in contexts where they are in sexual encounters or exposed to drugs.

Third, educators need to explore with students the social, psychological, and economic implications of the disease. This too can be a way to lower anxiety. By humanizing the epidemics, by letting students know how the disease has affected individuals and families, they may be more empathic to the needs and rights of persons infected with the HIV virus. Finally, education should provide information about community sources of assistance, not just on HIV infection but also on drug use, sexual behaviors, bereavement, and other areas touched by the epidemic.

This information needs to be sensitively presented in the context of ongoing educational relationships. Children and adolescents need to know teachers and counselors within each school they can approach for further information and clarification of concerns. AIDS awareness days with guest speakers may be very effective supplements to an educational program but they can never substitute for an ongoing program in HIV/AIDS education. In addition, other youth organizations such as Scouts or religious institutions may wish to develop their own programs of HIV/AIDS education and prevention.

For educational programs to be effective, three things are essential. First, there must be support and commitment from the highest levels of education. Second, there needs to be a consensus and commitment to move past present debates and teach comprehensive prevention strategies. Finally, this also requires a commitment to training administrators, guidance counselors, and both those presently in the field as well as those preparing to take their places in education.

Education for Individuals at Risk

Education cannot be limited to the schools. Certainly a key constituency in education has to be those involved in at-risk behaviors. This includes intravenous drug users and individuals who are sexually active, especially those practicing anal intercourse.

In many ways, gay advocacy organizations pioneered educational programs for at-risk groups. And, in fact, studies seem to indicate that gay sexual practices have changed in response to the HIV/AIDS epidemic (Schneider, 1988). Some of this educational material has been controversial because it offered graphic and explicit instructions for safer sex. Yet it is a model of the kinds of materials and education that will need to be produced and offered if HIV infection is to be inhibited. Tax monies are far more efficiently used for preventive activities that are effective than for treating newly infected cases. If preventive efforts in the United States toward those at risk for HIV infection through sexual contract are to be successful, a simple fact must be acknowledged. People are at risk because they are or are likely to be sexually active. At this point abstinence is not a likely alternative. Education, then, will have to discuss alternatives such as the use of condoms and safer sex in clear and frank terms. And this information should be presented in the broadest possible way—utilizing a variety of media including billboards, posters, and public service commercials. For example, in many European nations advertisements for condoms and messages about HIV prevention are common, appearing in rest rooms and subways. Similarly, condoms have to be readily accessible and inexpensive.

Educating IV drug users will be even more complex. Once in a famous flippant remark on the war in Vietnam, Vermont's Senator George Aiken suggested we declare victory and bring our troops home. In a sense that kind of thinking provides an alternative to our response to the drug war. We could declare victory and consider drug use a medical problem.

IV drug use remains a serious problem that may even worsen as persons begin to inject cocaine. It also becomes a major factor for the disease to spread more generally. For the duration of the epidemic, slowing the advance of the virus ought to be the primary public health goal. Alternatives to IV drug use such as methadone maintenance have been shown to reduce IV drug use and needle sharing (Ball et al., 1988). Such programs need to be expanded. Again, there needs to be explicit education aimed at IV drug users that offers accessible alternatives such as methadone maintenance, as well as suggested strategies for safer drug use and safer sex. More research needs to be done on other strategies such as needle distribution programs. But any programs that can be shown to be effective in reducing the spread of HIV infection ought be implemented.

Testing

After education, the next line of defense in the prevention of HIV infection lies in testing for the presence of the virus. It would be desirable if persons knew their status and acted responsibly in that knowledge.

Testing, then, should be easily accessible, confidential, and inexpensive. Mandatory testing is not likely to be effective for two reasons. First, the status of test results can readily change, especially in a relatively open society. The fact that one is HIV-negative at any one time does not mean that one will maintain that status. Mandatory and coercive testing is unlikely to be effective. As stated in previous sections only when the health of another is affected should testing be required. Naturally, testing will be most effective when supported by strong and enforced antidiscriminatory legislation.

For testing to be effective, it should be done in a context that emphasizes counseling. This is necessary for a number of reasons. Test results are not always as clear as they seem. At present the most common tests are the ELISA and Western blot test for antibodies to the HIV virus. Generally the ELISA test is used first. If the result is positive the person is generally tested again with the ELISA test. If a second positive is recorded a Western blot test is used to confirm the presence of antibodies.

This process attempts to minimize false positives, that is, persons who test positively for the virus even though the virus is not present. An initial positive result may not necessarily be confirmed in subsequent tests. Even if the person is HIV-positive, that person may not necessarily later develop the disease, nor is it predictable when the infection will produce symptoms of the disease.

A negative result, too, may have a number of meanings. It may mean that the person is not infected or it may simply mean that the antibodies, which may take up to 6 weeks to be produced, are not present. In the latter case someone may be infected even though he or she tests negative.

Counseling, then, becomes a critical adjunct to the testing process. In all cases, the person's motivations for taking the test ought to be explored. If there is evidence of at-risk behaviors, specific preventive strategies can be tailored to the individual. If there is an unrealistic obsession with the disease, for example, a person not evidently at risk insists on multiple tests, psychiatric referrals can be made because such obsessive behavior may be an indication of a compulsive disorder.

If the results are negative, the person may need to have those results interpreted and possibly, if evidence of exposure exists, have another test scheduled. In any case, there is opportunity to review with the person ways to eliminate or minimize future risk. This may be particularly critical because some persons who test negative may develop a false sense of invulnerability.

Should the results be positive, the person may need help in interpreting these results. The next section emphasizes the social and psychological needs of persons who are HIV-infected; here, it is important to mention that counseling at this level should at the very least help the person deal with their fears and anxieties, explore information about the HIV infection, and confront the ongoing dilemmas of sexual expression and drug use. This is critical if the person responds to the positive review by reacting in vengeful, hedonistic, or apathetic ways. He or she could infect others. In addition, the HIV-positive person immediately should consider treatment options.

Testing, then, should always be done in a context that allows counseling. This does not preclude innovative modes of testing. For example, mobile and street front units could offer confidential testing to transient populations such as runaway youth, the homeless, and drug users. Two new tests are currently being marketed; both at present do not offer actual home testing. In one test, blood is collected at home and sent to a laboratory. A few days later, an 800 number is called to get the result, using a private code number. If the results are positive, telephone counseling is provided. If the results are negative, no counseling is provided. This may be problematic, because counseling should be provided regardless of the result. A second "saliva" test actually tests mucosal material from the mouth and gums. Presently, this test is conducted at a doctor's office or clinic. Both procedures necessitate an evaluation of the effectiveness of phone counseling. Such an evaluation may provide a context for understanding the dilemmas presented by future technologies that truly allow home testing—that is, the interpretation of results by the tested person at home. On the one hand, these true at-home tests ensure accessable and confidential testing. On the other, they do not necessarily offer a supportive context for the interpretation of results. For that reason there ought to be continuing trials on the social and psychological implications of new testing procedures for the HIV virus.

CARE FOR THE INFECTED[1]

A life-threatening illness such as HIV infection is best perceived as consisting of a series of phases, each with its own particular issues and care needs. In HIV infection, the first phase, the prediagnostic phase, is characterized by the decision to undergo an HIV test. Often this is an important period to explore retrospectively. One can learn a great deal about a person's coping style and skills by examining the decision whether or not to take the test. First, it can reveal his or her knowledge and expectation about the disease. For example, in one case, a recovered IV drug user took the test when his dentist recognized pervasive thrush infection in his throat and mouth and suggested he had HIV infection. Despite the fact that the man was clearly at risk and had many symptoms of an impaired immune system such as evident swollen glands, night sweats, frequent illnesses, and thrush, he was convinced that the test would be negative. In addition to knowledge and beliefs about the disease, behaviors in this period will demonstrate characteristic ways of coping. In the previous case, for example, this young man frequently minimized and denied the threat of illness. Finally, this process can also illustrate important sources of social support. One may find out with whom the person discussed the decision to take the test or the results.

It is important to acknowledge that many individuals will take the HIV test for a number of reasons, including as a requirement for insurance, travel to foreign countries that require documentation of HIV status, beginning a new relationship, concerns about possible risk, and even as a routine medical test. Counselors are well advised, then, to explore motivations for testing as well.

The next phase, the acute phase, is the period in which one learns that one has a diagnosis of life-threatening illness. That period, briefly discussed in the last section, is often a period of intense crisis. Here the individual must make a series of decisions—medical, psychological, interpersonal, spiritual—about how, at least initially, to cope with this crisis.

[1]Doka (1993) offered an extensive discussion of managing a life-threatening illness. This section summarizes material from that work. In addition, Winiarski (1991) provided an excellent treatment of AIDS-related psychotherapy.

Counseling at this period, beginning with the test results and beyond, must consider a series of issues. The infected individual needs to understand the disease, particularly the health risks they may impart to others. This is particularly critical because the individual may have few manifest indications of illness.

Infected individuals also should develop strategies to deal with issues created by the disease. Three issues are primary. First, individuals need to consider the issue of disclosure—who they will tell of their illness. In a disease such as HIV infection that generates such a strong sense of fear and stigma, often individuals will seek to carefully control information about their condition. This protectiveness is understandable. But it does limit their support. As they begin to experience symptoms, attempts at withholding information can be counterproductive. Most importantly, others around them may have been or may continue to be at risk, creating a context where counselors may have a duty to warn. The duty to warn, established by the court case *Tarasoff v. Regents of the University of California*, places counselors in a difficult position. There is a tension between the duty to warn others at risk and confidentiality. As Winiarski (1991) notes, this tension can be abated if the therapist emphasizes prevention and can work with the partner. When this is impossible, the partner's identity is known, and the client refuses to use unsafe practices, the therapist, after extensive (and documented) discussion with colleagues and supervisors, may determine that it is necessary to breach confidentiality.

A second issue that infected persons may need to consider is treatment options. They need to explore with physicians their options for both when to begin treatments as well as the advantages and disadvantages of various therapies. At the very least infected individuals may wish to examine and improve their own health and lifestyle practices.

It may also be important to consider various life consequences at this point. The course of HIV infection is both complex and unpredictable. Many persons may remain asymptomatic for years. However, others may begin to experience illness more quickly, especially if a test takes place comparatively late in the course of the infection. Then, too, the course of the disease is varied. Some individuals may experience mental disorientation, confusion, or mental illness. In fact close to 68% of persons with HIV infection are likely to experience some degree of dementia or other psychiatric illness as the disease progresses (Rundell et al., 1988; Schofferman, 1988). At the earliest points in the illness, then, it is helpful if individuals consider such issues as power of attorney or advance directives. If they are parents, they need to develop permanancy plans for their offspring.

In addition, there are other contingencies that may be considered. Infected persons may need to decide whether or not they should continue on their job. If they are employed and have medical insurance, the issue of continued insurability should be considered.

There may be other issues that infected persons may need to consider in the acute phase. These can include examining their internal strengths and limitations; considering other resources, vitality, feelings, and fears; and considering the ways the illness may affect future plans and relationships with others.

After the crisis of diagnosis is passed, infected persons move into the chronic phase. In this phase an individual is struggling both with the disease and its treatment. One of the promising aspects in HIV/AIDS is that the chronic phase continues to be gradually lengthened. In fact, there is some hope that future treatments will allow a greater control of the disease, letting infected persons live decades longer. In HIV infection, persons usually are asymptomatic at the beginning of this period. The illness later is characterized by cycles of opportunistic illnesses and partial or complete recovery. As the illness continues, the immune system is likely to be more impaired. Often at this period the health and treatment regimen is more complex, the illness more pervasive, and the recovery more partial. Throughout this time, infected individuals have to cope with life's other demands, including work and/or school. Often there is an attempt to live as reasonably normal a life as possible within the confines of the disease and its treatment.

There are a number of issues that persons may have to deal with at this point in the illness. Two of the most critical are managing symptoms and side effects and carrying out health and treatment regimens. This is particularly complicated in HIV infection for a number of reasons. The disease itself is complex and unpredictable. The treatment can be expensive and complicated. Medication may not lead to immediate or dramatic improvements or even have visible effects, discouraging adherence. The present lack of a cure may also weaken motivation. And when there are other complications in life, such as crises of homelessness or other losses, adherence can become problematic.

Caregivers can be helpful to persons struggling with these issues. First, infected individuals may need someone to listen to their concerns about the disease and treatment. In some cases caregivers may encourage individuals to take more active roles in their treatment, assisting them in explaining concerns to their physicians. In other cases, caregivers may themselves need to advocate, especially when clients do not feel self-empowered. Second, caregivers can help identify individuals, circumstances, or strategies that inhibit adherence to medication and treatment protocols. And, third, caregivers can help infected individuals to explore any decisions they may make to seek alternate therapies. When these therapies offer no harm and they are complementary to traditional therapies (e.g., vitamins, diet, imagery), they should not be discouraged. For these therapies may aid adherence to the medical regimen and allow the individual to reassert a sense of control so challenged by the disease. In other circumstances, an individual may choose to refuse conventional treatment and/or engage in nonconventional and noncomplementary therapies. Competent adults retain the right to refuse treatment. In this case, it is the counselor's role to assist the individual in obtaining information that may influence treatment decisions as well as to help him or her explore the risks and benefits of that refusal. It is also appropriate for the counselor to assess competency, because HIV infection can manifest itself in dementia and other psychiatric symptoms.

Counseling may help the infected individual deal with other issues inherent in the chronic phase. Caregivers can assist individuals in managing stress and examining the ways that they are coping with the illness. Aiding individuals to prevent and manage medical crises can also reaffirm a sense of control and raise morale. Other areas that may be explored include helping infected individuals to maximize support, preserve self-concept, ventilate feelings and fears, and find final meaning in the experience of illness. It is also critical for individuals to try to normalize life in the midst of disease. This means examining the ways that the disease affects roles and relationships. Naturally this will involve discussion of sexual relationships. Because HIV infection can be spread through sexual acts, counselors will need to encourage infected individuals to share information about the disease with prospective sexual partners as well as to discuss safer sex alternatives. Throughout the chronic phase, an infected individual will struggle with a variety of losses, such as losses of hope, self-esteem, motivation and interest, security, sexual freedom, privacy, community, health, and meaning—all of which need to be explored (Nord, 1997).

Counselors may also assume the role of case manager or advocate and train others for this role. The role of case manager is multifaceted and essentially involves coordinating an array of services that allow the client to function optimally. Case managers may monitor medical treatment, assist with formal bureaucracies, and assist other caregivers in better utilizing available services. Some advocacy groups, such as Gay Men's Health Crisis, routinely provide case management services, as do many hospitals. When these sources of help are not so readily available, the counselor with a knowledge of available resources and a strong relationship with the client may assume this role.

In the terminal phase of the disease the infected individual faces the crisis of death. The medical goal now shifts. It is no longer to extend life but rather to provide the individual comfort.

As the caregivers work with persons in these phases, it is critical that the dying person set the tone for conversation. Weisman (1972) reminds us that individuals who are dying often have "middle knowledge"; that is, they drift in and out of the awareness of dying. In this phase individuals also have to deal with certain issues and tasks. Among them are:

1. dealing with symptoms, discomfort, pain, and incapacitation,
2. managing health and institutional procedures,
3. managing stress and examining coping,
4. dealing effectively with caregivers,
5. preparing for death and saying good-bye,
6. preserving relationships with family and friends,
7. preserving self-concept,
8. ventilating feelings and fears, and
9. finding meaning in life and death.

In addition to these tasks, individuals who are dying may need to make certain decisions regarding their treatment or care. They may need to consider whether and when to enter a hospice program and if so what type of hospice program. Although hospice programs can provide excellent palliative care, they may not be appropriate for everyone in the terminal phase. Many hospice programs require the participation of a primary caregiver. In other cases, persons may not be psychologically capable of admitting that the goal is now palliative. Finally, many hospice programs are home based. For some dying at home may not be an appropriate option.

If dying persons have not already made decisions regarding termination of treatment, it may be helpful if they are willing to discuss their wishes as to when and under what circumstances they would wish treatment to continue or cease. And it may be helpful to designate an individual who would have durable power of attorney, allowing him or her to make decisions when the individual who is dying is no longer capable of making his or her wishes known. Such statements of intent can be very helpful particularly in cases of AIDS. Because many of the opportunistic infections are treatable, it may be difficult to know when and what interventions should cease. Given the fact that symptoms of AIDS can include dementia and other psychiatric manifestations, these decisions should be discussed early in the illness and reviewed throughout its course. If an individual has openly stated his or her wishes and has the support of family and significant others, his or her choice is more likely to be respected.

HIV/AIDS is a disease that has become dreaded and has further stigmatized already marginalized groups. Because of this, caregivers have to actively seek to develop and build trusts. Many infected persons may scrutinize caregivers' behaviors to see whether they disapprove of either their disease or their lifestyle. Effective caregivers, then, need to convey both in their verbal and nonverbal behaviors honesty, nonjudgmental acceptance, and a respect for the person that encourages that individual to become a partner in treatment.

It is also important for caregivers to recognize the particular problems of each of the HIV-infected populations. For example, IV drug users who are HIV-infected often experience multiple problems. Many have a low income and may lack housing, insurance, and social support. As they struggle with the disease they may also grapple with addiction, alternating between cycles of recovery from substance use and relapse. They may present intense problems for medical management of the disease. They may have strong coping mechanisms of denial, denying both addiction and disease. A strong orientation to the present often makes adherence to a medical regimen as well as preventive actions difficult. In addition, there is always the danger that infected individuals may continue or relapse into drug use as a way of coping with the illness. And there is another potential problem. IV drug users may have multiple members of their families simultaneously struggling with the disease, reflecting both patterns of infection (e.g., an infected wife or children) as well as a history of shared drug use.

HIV-infected women, too, have distinct issues. At present most of the women in the United States who have AIDS contracted the disease through IV drug use or sex with an infected partner. As a result women with HIV infection tend to be women of color as well as low income. Women account for a small percentage of HIV/AIDS infection in the United States (Richardson, 1988). Therefore their unique concerns are often overlooked. In Africa, however, women account for approximately half the cases of HIV infection. As addressed in an earlier chapter, the nature of the disease tends to vary in women. One of the major issues may involve the care of children both when the women are ill as well as permanancy planning should the women die. Infected women may also need counseling to evaluate decisions on whether or not to continue a pregnancy. Caregivers need to acknowledge that such decisions are quite complex. There is a risk that the child will be born HIV-infected. In addition, the mother's ability to care for the child may be constrained by the illness. The treatment of the illness will be complicated by the pregnancy. However, many of these women may have strong religious and cultural beliefs about terminating a pregnancy. The child, too, may be perceived as an affirmation of life as well as a legacy.

Gay men represent a major population of HIV-infected persons in the United States. It is an extremely heterogeneous population spanning all races, religions, and income groups. Caregivers need to be sensitive to these differences as well as to other variations in this population such as degree of openness about sexuality, acceptance of their sexuality by their biological families, and level of participation and identification with the larger gay community. Caregivers should also exhibit a sensitivity to the chosen family, that is, those persons within the patient's intimate network. One of the devastating aspects of the HIV/AIDS epidemic is the degree to which the gay community has been devastated. It is not unusual, then, that someone may be struggling not only with his own illness but also with the illness of so many within his intimate network.

Children who are infected with HIV also experience not only a distinct medical syndrome but various psychosocial problems as well. In the early years of the epidemic, children were infected by blood or blood products, such as those used in the treatment of hemophilia or prenatally. In recent years prenatal infection has become the predominant mode of infection. Again this amplifies the multiple risks and crises experienced by these children. They are disproportionately lower income and children of color. Because their mothers are either struggling with disease and possibly addiction or have died, many of these children are in foster care, sometimes with extended family members.

In treating children with HIV infection, it is important to recognize that the child's developmental state will influence the ways he or she copes with the illness. This is complicated because many HIV-infected children are also likely to have developmental deficiencies. Because many of these children have been infected perinatally, many of their mothers are likely to have been IV drug users. Their children are likely to suffer from fetal drug syndrome and other ongoing developmental deficiencies. In fact, a positive HIV result at birth, whether or not the child seroreverts, is an excellent predictor of subsequent developmental difficulties. Thus, these children may demonstrate behavioral, cognitive, affective, and physical development inappropriate for their chronological age.

Children at each age, though, are likely to experience many problems. Infants infected with HIV often show a failure to thrive. Many of the children who do not serorevert will die of AIDS in infancy. In the first 2 years, there are a number of ways that life-threatening illness affects the infant. The intermittent periods of separation, the ever-changing environment, as well as painful and (to the infant) incomprehensible procedures may impair both the child's bonding and his or her development of trust. Parental bonding too may be affected in these first years by the state of parental health, concerns of foster families as to whether the child will remain in their care, and medical uncertainty as to whether or not the child will serorevert. Periods of hospitalization can be particularly frightening because an infant may feel abandoned to strangers who cause pain. Hospital programs that allow unlimited visitation by caregivers, including overnight stays, and encourage full parental participation in care and medication often mitigate some of the separation anxiety and isolation that children may experience during hospitalization and facilitate parental bonding.

As the child continues to age and develop, the physical limitations caused by the disease and its treatments, as well as parental restrictions and overprotectiveness, may limit his or her ability to explore the world and develop autonomy. In addition, parental attempts to set limits and provide discipline, so critical at this stage, may be compromised by concern about the illness. Caregivers may be anxious and overly restrictive, sympathetically lenient, or seemingly inconsistent and arbitrary (if discipline is based upon an assessment of the child's condition at that time). The result is that the child's developmental tasks of both exploring the environment and finding and recognizing limits are impaired.

While the child's ability to understand the reality of death or of life-threatening illness is a topic debated by many professionals, the differences between the adult's and the child's understanding of the situation as well as the anxiety generated in caregivers and children by the illness can complicate communication between the caregivers and their child. Caregivers may have considerable uncertainty about how, how much, and when to respond to their child's questions. The young child too may have considerable misunderstanding of the nature, cause, and treatment of the illness. Again, the mortality rate is high because these children's immune system is too compromised to fight childhood infections. Almost 30% of HIV-infected children who were infected perinatally die between the ages of 2 and 5 (Mann et al., 1992).

Perinatally HIV-infected children who survive to age 5 and start school must contend with four problems. First, developmental disabilities due to the prenatal environment can impair subsequent school performance. Second, the illness and treatment can retard intellectual development, particularly if side effects include lethargy or confusion. Third, the treatment regimen may be difficult to manage within the classroom environment. Fourth, teachers may be fearful of dealing with an HIV-infected child. Nonetheless, Public Law 94-142 clearly affirms the rights of

HIV-positive children to educational evaluation and placement in the least restrictive, appropriate, educational setting. In school systems with little experience with HIV infection, physicians may need to act as both advocates and educators.

Schools thrust the ill child into interaction with healthy peers, which can create other issues. The stigma of the illness, limitations on activity, lack of self-confidence, and low self-esteem are but a few of the problems that can arise. In some cases other parents, afraid of the disease and overly protective of their own children, may discourage or prohibit their children from playing with the ill child, especially if they suspect HIV infection. Caregivers may wish to consider the advantages of education programs designed for HIV-infected children. However, although such schools can have increased sensitivity to the child's needs, they may limit the child's opportunities to interact with well peers and reinforce a sense of stigma.

The illness complicates the struggles for mastery and independence typical of this age. Parents may be reluctant to allow their child necessary autonomy, thereby breeding overdependence. The child's own ability to master his or her environment may be affected either by the direct limitations of the disease or by an impaired self-concept. On the other hand, caregivers can utilize this natural desire for mastery, particularly within the chronic phase, by encouraging the child's increased responsibility and participation in treatment and treatment decisions. As the child reaches adolescence, there may be additional concerns about sexual activity.

In summation, HIV infection is a complex syndrome demanding careful medical monitoring. However, even more than that it requires a sensitivity that can challenge caregivers. In a context characterized by stigma and fear, caregivers will need to provide clear reassurance that the dread that accompanies the disease finds no home with them.

CREATING A HUMANE SYSTEM

The Role of Public Health

One of the critical roles of public health in the HIV/AIDS paradigm will be "decathexizing" the epidemic. By that it is meant that public health agencies should take a significant role in education and advocacy that will reduce the levels of both fear and stigma associated with that disease. C. Everett Koop, the Surgeon General in the Reagan administration, filled that role admirably, educating the public about the disease while maintaining a compassionate and non-judgmental attitude toward all those that are infected. The surgeon general—in fact, even the president—should be conscious of symbolic opportunities that will allow the decathexizing of the disease. For example, hosting HIV-positive children during the Easter egg hunt at the White House would be a wonderful way to demonstrate both the normalcy of HIV-positive persons as well as to make a statement about irrational fear of HIV-infected persons.

Beyond the critical symbolic role, public health agencies throughout the country need to take an active role in combating the epidemic. This would include a broad role in public health education. In addition, public health agencies should make convenient and confidential testing a priority. Even anonymous testing ought to be an available option. It is, however, clearly less desirable because it limits any counseling prior to and after testing. For testing to be successful, public health agencies should advocate for HIV-positive persons, working to ease discrimination against persons who are HIV-positive and advocating for supportive services. Treatment that is humane rather than punitive will encourage testing. Other roles will need to be assessed locally. For example, in areas where there is a low prevalence of seropositivity, contact tracing may be acceptable.

In addition, public health agencies may encourage health care workers in general to use universal precautions and to provide compassionate care. Public health agencies, then, should take a leading role in providing appropriate education on the medical, psychosocial, and spiritual needs of persons who are HIV-positive. They can also offer emotional support and ongoing education to health care workers.

Approximately 150 years ago, public health agencies helped stem the cholera epidemic. A hundred years ago, they played a critical role in preventing the spread of tuberculosis. This new epidemic provides yet another opportunity for public health agencies to engage in a leadership role.

The Response of the Health Care System

It is not only public health agencies that will be challenged by the HIV/AIDS epidemic. The entire health care system will be stressed. In a sense, the HIV/AIDS epidemic has come at a very inappropriate time. AIDS involves expensive and complex medical management. It comes at a time when there is a real concern with cutting and containing costs. Especially with more economically marginal groups such as IV drug users, there is a danger that care can be less than adequate.

Yet there are innovative models and effective systems in place to care for populations who are chronically ill. In areas where large numbers of persons are infected, specialized services may be developed. For example, in New York City the Gay Men's Health Crisis has had a significant role in providing an array of supportive services to infected individuals such as home care, support groups, assistance with medication, and advocacy. Developing partnerships with such groups makes considerable sense. Such agencies often have credibility with infected individuals who may be more suspicious of other agencies. In addition such agencies can often provide culturally sensitive services. As such agencies develop they can extend their services to other groups as well. For example, the Gay Men's Health Crisis initially offered services primarily to gay men. Now it serves other groups as well.

In other areas with a lesser concentration of HIV-infected persons such specialized services both are unlikely to develop and may not be cost effective. However, most areas have a system already developed to support older persons with chronic conditions living at home. This gerontological network may have to reframe its mission, emphasizing its ability to offer services that provide a continuum of care for individuals who are chronically ill. In all areas the gerontological network, including nursing homes, may have a critical role in providing some level of supportive care.

Hospices also have been challenged by the HIV epidemic. In the past two decades, the hospice movement has undergone phenomenal growth. Hospice, though, was initially developed to provide symptom control and pain relief to individuals in the terminal phase of cancer. Medically, the terminal phase of AIDS is complex and creates distinct issues for palliation. Hospice staff, then, will need continued training and support to master the new knowledge that AIDS palliation will require. There are other issues as well. In many cases hospice care depends on a primary care person, or a familial caregiver in the home. In many cases person dying of AIDS may have seen their families, friends, and intimate networks decimated by the disease. There may not be caregivers, or at least well caregivers, left. There may be management problems as well. For example, persons with AIDS who have engaged in IV drug use or who are living in homes with drug users may misuse pain medications. Such persons may experience a variety of other problems. They may be homeless or come from problematic environments.

There are other issues as well. The caregiving community, especially in hospice, is largely White and middle class, as are many of its volunteers. Hospice programs often depend on volunteers who may be reluctant to be involved with AIDS cases or to travel to lower income communities where many persons with AIDS reside.

These problems are not unsolvable. But they will require training, funding, and support. They also will necessitate models of care that move beyond the present home care system. For example, in San Francisco, the gay community has developed an extensive buddy system that enables persons to receive hospice care in their own homes even if there is not a primary caregiver. Hospices serving IV drug users have developed special residences or mobile teams that can medicate daily.

In many ways there is real value in involving systems such as the gerontological and hospice communities. These systems provide critical care and service. But they do more than that. By engaging larger communities and volunteers, by providing training even to those who may not eventually work with HIV-positive persons, they provide a cadre of professionals and volunteers who can help to prevent the disease and to dissipate the fear that it has created.

CARE FOR THE AFFECTED

Care has to be provided not only to those infected with the disease but also to those who are affected by it. The very nature of the HIV epidemic magnifies and complicates the issue of bereavement in the Western world. Until the epidemic, the death rate was highest among the elderly. Most AIDS-related deaths take place among younger populations. This has two implications.

First, the deaths of elderly persons in the United States and other industrialized nations are developmentally expected. By that it is meant that the death of an older person, although it can cause great grief, does not shatter one's expectations about death. When a younger person dies, the death is perceived as out of the natural order. This often leaves survivors feeling more vulnerable and can intensify grief reactions.

These reactions can vary and may include physical, cognitive, affective, behavioral, and spiritual responses. Among very common reactions are anger, anxiety, and guilt. Anger may be directed at a number of sources including those held responsible for infection, as well as the government or medical system for perceived inaction or inhumanity. It may be a spiritual anger, directed at God. Or the anger may target the person who died, either for abandoning the survivors or for lifestyle factors that may have led to infection. Guilt is also a common reaction of bereaved survivors. They may feel guilty about the quality of the relationship, feel that they have contributed to the death directly or indirectly, and perhaps feel a moral guilt—that this death is a punishment for their failures. Anxiety may also be heightened, especially for those involved in intimate and sexual relationships with the deceased.

A second factor that affects AIDS-related deaths is that because this population is younger their deaths are likely to affect a larger population than the elderly. By the time an older person dies, they may be more disengaged from others. Friends and family may have predeceased them. They are retired from work roles. Younger persons are likely to leave comparatively more bereaved family members and friends to grieve.

Yet the fact that this is an epidemic may also mean that survivors themselves are coping with multiple losses. This is especially true among families of hemophiliacs, gay communities, or communities characterized by heavy IV drug use. For example, one gay funeral director in San Francisco shared that though he was only approaching 40 years of age, he had survived more than 50 friends and acquaintances that were his age or younger. Similarly, families troubled by IV drug use may experience multigenerational loss.

In addition to these difficulties, AIDS-related deaths are often disenfranchised. Disenfranchised grief comes in response to losses that are not socially supported, publicly mourned, or openly acknowledged (Doka, 1989). Grief can be disenfranchised for four major reasons, all of which are evident in the AIDS-related deaths. First, grief can be disenfranchised because the relationship is not recognized. In the United States and many other Western nations, relationships between kin are socially validated. When one loses a family member, there is an acknowledgment that one has a right to grieve that loss. However, other persons may be involved in close, intimate relationships. Yet because these relationships do not have social standing within the larger community, grief may be unacknowledged by others. Gay lovers and friends, the lovers of IV drug users, foster parents and siblings, coworkers, and even corrections officers guarding HIV-positive inmates represent examples of the types of person who may be deeply affected by the death of a person with AIDS. Yet their loss may be unacknowledged by others.

A second category of disenfranchised grief is where the loss is unacknowledged by others. Often this refers to non-death-related losses such as divorce, job loss, or infertility. But it can also refer to losses that others simply do not recognize or consider as creating grief. Losses experienced in the course of illness, especially when someone manifests AIDS-related dementia, may be an example of this condition. Here the person is still alive, but others may grieve the absence of the person they once knew. In addition, children who go in and out of foster care while their HIV-infected parents are hospitalized will also experience grief.

Grief can also be disenfranchised when the griever is considered incapable of expressing grief. Very young children and persons with developmental disabilities may exhibit their grief in different ways, but that does not mean they do not experience that loss. Again, the HIV epidemic will leave many bereaved children, some with developmental delays.

Finally, there are disenfranchising deaths. These are deaths that are so stigmatized that grievers are reluctant to share their loss with others. Some victim-precipitated homicides or suicides may leave survivors feeling so guilty and ashamed that they are reluctant to reach out for support. AIDS-related deaths also carry a similar stigma. I think of one 15-year-old boy whose older brother, whom he deeply loved, died of AIDS. When asked if he could discuss his loss with his peers, he responded in shocked tones. "Are you kidding? I do not want any of my friends to even know I had a brother." His self-protectiveness is understandable. Yet the cost is high as he bears his pain alone.

The challenge to caregivers in the HIV epidemic will be to enfranchise disenfranchised grievers. This will involve validating and acknowledging the grief that persons are experiencing. Grief counselors will need a sensitivity to all the nuances of loss that persons may experience in both the course and the aftermath of the illness. They will also need to respect the many dimensions of loss.

It also seems clear that making grief counseling readily accessible will be critical. Studies of the gay community have shown long-lasting deleterious psychological distress for AIDS-related bereavement that is lengthy and complicated by multiple losses (Martin, 1988; Martin & Dean, 1993; Viney, Henry, Walker and Crooks, 1992). Studies of communities affected by IV drug use or of the orphans of the epidemic, many of whom may have suffered multiple losses of family members, likely would yield similar results.

Finding ways to make bereavement counseling accessible will be a challenge on many levels. First, there will need to be a mechanism to provide for funding counseling services. Bereavement counseling, especially because it will affect the health and well being of survivors, should be covered in any health care reform. In the United States, the current emphasis on managed care creates difficulty for counselors. While organizations will need to encompass bereavement counseling, counselors may need to explore different models of counseling, such as timing and pacing the counseling throughout the grieving process, to address the cost containment goals of managed care.

The accessibility of counseling, though, refers to more than simply issues of finances. Considerable research and training will be needed to ensure that counselors are sensitive to the unique issues created by HIV infection. This includes the issue of cultural sensitivity. For example, in working with survivors of IV drug users, counselors need to know something about drug use and to be sensitive to the strains of low income life. In working with families of color, it also is essential that counselors understand the cultures of each group, emphasizing and exploring the ways that each culture and class facilitates or complicates the grieving process. Similarly, in working with survivors within the gay community, counselors need to know something about the history of the gay movement to understand the multiple losses, such as the losses of sexual freedom and community, experienced by gays. In addition, counselors must be sensitive to the different ranges of relationships that exist within the gay community. As Nord (1997) notes, families of choice do not have the same range of terms (e.g., "aunt" or "cousin") that denote kin-based relationships. Other cultures, too, may understand relationships differently or provide for significant roles such as "godchild" or "godparent" that may be overlooked. Counselors are wise, then, to identify the intimate networks that exist around the deceased and indicate in their materials that all survivors touched by the life of the deceased will be affected by the death. Support groups that specify lovers, spouses, or family may unintentionally exclude grievers.

Finally, attempts to provide counseling and support need to encompass caregivers. The HIV epidemic provides unique stressors on caregivers. They are dealing with clients, often culturally diverse populations, that are likely to be their age or younger. In many cases, they may treat patients for years, developing strong bonds. The unpredictable nature of the disease complicates both treatment and management. All of these factors have been known to increase occupational stress (Vachon, 1987). In addition, caregivers' own grief may be disenfranchised by others, by their own sense of their professional roles, or by a reluctance, either theirs or others, to discuss grief.

Medical and health organizations will have to respond creatively to the needs of their caregivers. This may involve providing training or stress management.

But it is more than an individual problem. Organizations will need to provide ongoing inservice and strong support through support groups and team building experiences. Organizations will often need to validate the grief of caregivers and provide opportunities for them to mourn, perhaps by occasional memorial services or varied rituals when favorite clients die. The alternative is higher attrition, absenteeism, lower morale, and an environment characterized by signs of caregiver stress such as displaced anger and hostility. In the beleaguered health community such sensitivity may seem difficult to achieve.

CONCLUSION: DECATHEXIZING THE EPIDEMIC

As mentioned earlier, the key to creating a humane future lies in decathexizing the epidemic. As long as HIV infection continues to generate the fear, loathing, and dread that it has historically spawned, it will be difficult to treat the disease. As long as a disease engenders such dread, a number of deleterious effects are evident. First, policies are likely to be driven more by fear than by realistic attempts to rationally control the disease. Second, persons with the infection themselves become sources of dread, dehumanizing treatment. When this occurs, infected individuals are reluctant to come forward, fearful of revealing a perceived stigma. This then inhibits identification and treatment.

Decathexizing a dreaded disease is, of course, difficult. At the very least, it involves HIV education rooted in the context of health education (so as not to further isolate the disease), at all educational levels. But it also involves depoliticizing the disease and creating a context where the media, in all its many forms, presents AIDS as a disease, rather than a mark of membership in one group or another. That level of restraint, in a democratic system, is hard to achieve. There is a call, then, for leadership of all sectors—political, religious, educational, medical, and scientific—to encourage that restraint and nourish that compassion.

In the end, dreaded diseases have shown humans at both their most heroic and their most venal. They have demonstrated fear and avarice. They have amplified human divisions and magnified human cruelty. But they have also demonstrated the human capacity for caring and compassion. The critical element is to remember, even in the midst of fear in crisis, that the enemy is a parasitic virus and not one another.

BIBLIOGRAPHY

Adam, B. (1992). Sociology and people: Living with AIDS. In J. Huber & B. Schneider (Eds.), *The social context of AIDS* (pp. 3–18). Newbury Park, CA: Sage.

AHA says fear of AIDS goes too far. (1984). *RN, 47,* 13.

AIDS and drug addiction in New York. (1989, September/October). *The Futurist,* 7.

AIDS and entrepreneurs. (1991). *Hastings Center Report, 21*(6), 2–3.

Aires, P. (1987). *The hour of our death.* New York: Knopf.

Allen, J. R., & Curren, J. W. (1988). Prevention of AIDS and HIV infection: Needs and priorities for epidemiologic research. *American Journal of Public Health, 78,* 381–386.

Altman, D. (1986). *AIDS in the mind of America.* Garden City, NY: Doubleday.

Altman, D. (1988). Legitimation through disaster: AIDS and the gay movement. In E. Fee & D. Fox (Eds.), *AIDS: The burden of history* (pp. 301–315). Berkeley, CA: University of California Press.

Anderson, W. (1991). The New York needle trial: The politics of public health in the age of AIDS. *American Journal of Public Health, 81,* 1506–1517.

Ball, J. C., Longe, R. W., Myers, P. C., & Friedman, S. (1988). Reducing the risk of AIDS through methadone maintenance treatment. *Journal of Health and Social Behavior, 29,* 214–226.

Barnett, T., & Blaikie, P. (1992). *AIDS in Africa: Its present and future impact.* New York: Guilford Press.

Batchelor, W. (1988). AIDS 1988: The science and the limits of science. *American Psychology, 43,* 853–858.

Bayer, R. (1989). *Private acts, social consequences: AIDS and the politics of public health.* New York: Free Press.

Beauchamp, D. (1986, December). Morality and the health of the body politic. *Hastings Center Report,* 30–36.

Becker, H. S. (1963). *Outsiders: Studies in the sociology of deviance.* New York: Free Press.

Benjamin, A. E., & Lee, P. R. (1988). Public policy: Federalism and AIDS. *Death Studies, 12,* 573–595.

Berk, R. (Ed.). (1988). *The social impact of AIDS in the U.S.* Cambridge, MA: Abt.

Beveridge, W. (1977). *Influenza: The last great plague.* New York: Prodist.

Boaz, D. (1994, September 10). Op-ed. *New York Times,* p. I:19:4.

Boccaccio, G. (1978). Plague in Siena: An Italian chronicle. In W. Bowsky (Ed.), *The Black Death: A turning point in history?* (pp. 13–14). Huntington, NY: Krieger.

Boen, W. (1981). Changing patterns of ideas about disease. In H. Rothschild (Ed.), *Biocultural aspects of disease* (pp. 25–93). New York: Academic Press.

Boswell, J. (1980). *Christianity, social intolerance and homosexuality.* Chicago: University of Chicago Press.

Bowsky, W. (Ed.). (1978). *The Black Death: A turning point in history?* Huntington, NY: Krieger.

Brandt, A. (1977). *No magic bullet: A social history of venereal disease in the United States since 1880.* New York: Oxford University Press.

Brandt, A. (1988a). AIDS and metaphor: Toward the social meaning of epidemic disease. *Social Research, 55,* 413–432.

Brandt, A. (1988b). AIDS in historical perspective: Four lessons from the history of sexually transmitted diseases. *American Journal of Public Health, 781,* 367–371.

Brandt, A. (1988c). The syphilis epidemic and its relation to AIDS. *Science, 239,* 375–380.

Braun, A. (1977). *The story of cancer: Its nature, causes and control.* Reading, MA: Addison-Wesley.

Brieux, E. (1913). *Damaged goods* (J. Pollack, Trans.). New York: Brentano's.

Brody, S. N. (1974). *The disease of the soul: Leprosy in medieval literature.* Ithaca, NY: Cornell University Press.

Brown, P. (1991). Conflict rages over alternative AIDS theories. *New Scientist, 132,* 9–10.

Bull, C., & Morales, J. (1995, January 24). Crisis in Cuba. *The Advocate,* p. 1.

Campbell, A. M. (1966). *The Black Death and men of learning.* New York: AMS Press.

Campbell, J. (with Bill Moyers). (1988). *The power of myth.* New York: Doubleday.

Centers for Disease Control. (1981, June 5). Pneumocystis carinii pneumonia in Los Angeles. *Morbidity and Mortality Weekly Report,* pp. 250–252.

Check, W. (1985, August). Public education on AIDS: Not only the media's responsibility. *Hastings Center Report,* 27–31.

Claster, J. (1982). *The medieval experience: 300–1400.* New York: New York University Press.

Coates, T. J., Stous, R., Kegeles, S., Lo, B., Mores, S., & McKusick, L. (1988). AIDS antibody testing: Will it stop the AIDS epidemic? Will it help people infected with HIV? *American Psychology, 43,* 859–864.

Cohen, A. K. (1966). *Deviance and control.* Englewood Cliffs, NJ: Prentice-Hall.

Cohen, F. (1995). Epidemiology of HIV infection and AIDS in children. In F. Cohen & J. Durham (Eds.), *Women, children and HIV/AIDS* (pp. 137–155). New York: Springer.

Cohen, F., & Durham, J. (1993). *Women, children and HIV/AIDS.* New York: Springer.

Cohen, I., & Elder, A. (1989). Major cities and disease crises: A comparative perspective. *Social Science History, 13,* 29–63.

Cornish, E. (1986). Farewell, sexual revolution. Hello, new Victorianism. *The Futurist, 20*(1), 2, 49.

Crosby, A. (1976). *Epidemic and peace, 1918.* Westport, CT: Greenwood Press.

Crosby, A. (1977). The pandemic of 1918. In J. Osborn (Ed.), *Influenza in America, 1918–1976* (pp. 5–14). New York: Prodist.

Curtis, T. (1992, March 19). The origins of AIDS. *Rolling Stone,* 54–60, 106–108.

Dalton, H. (1989). AIDS in blackface. *Daedalus, 118*(3), 205–227.

Defoe, D. (1911). *Journal of the plague years.* New York: E. P. Dutton.

Delaporte, F. (1986). *Disease and civilization: The cholera in Paris 1832.* Cambridge, MA: MIT Press.

Des Jarlais, D., Casriel, C., & Friedman, S. (1988). The new death among IV drug users. In I. Corless & M. Pittman Lindeman (Eds.), *AIDS: Principles, practices and politics* (pp. 135–150). New York: Hemisphere.

Des Jarlais, D., & Friedman, S. (1988). The psychology of preventing AIDS among intravenous drug users: A social learning conceptualization. *American Psychology, 43,* 865–870.

Des Jarlais, D., Friedman, S., Casriel, C., & Kott, A. (1987). AIDS and preventing initiation into intravenous (IV) drug use. *Psychology and Health, 1,* 179–194.

Des Jarlais, D., & Stephenson, B. (1991). History, ethics, and politics in AIDS prevention research. *American Journal of Public Health, 81,* 1393–1394.

De Tocqueville, A. (1945). *Democracy in America* (H. Reeve text rev. by F. Bowen & P. Bradley). New York: Knopf. (Original work published 1835)

Doka, K. J. (1989). *Disenfranchised grief: Recognizing hidden sorrow.* Lexington, MA: Lexington Books.

Doka, K. J. (1993). *Living with life-threatening illness: A guide for patients, their families, and caregivers.* Lexington, MA: Lexington Press.

Douglas, M. (1970). *National symbols: Explorations in cosmology.* New York: Random House.

Dubos, R., & Dubos, J. (1952). *The white plague: Tuberculosis, man and society.* Boston: Little, Brown.

Duesberg, P. (1988). HIV is not the cause of AIDS. *Science, 241,* 514.

Duesberg, P. (1995). Is HIV the cause of AIDS? *Lancet, 346,* 1371–1372.

Durey, M. (1979). *The return of the plague: British society and the cholera 1831–1832.* Dublin, Ireland: Gill & MacMillan.

Eckholm, E. (1985, September 12). Poll finds many AIDS fears that experts say are groundless. *New York Times,* p. II:11:3.

Faltz, B., & Madover, S. (1987). Treatment of substance abuse in patients with HIV infection. *Advances in Alcohol and Substance Abuse, 7,* 143–157.

Farmer, P., & Klienman, A. (1989). AIDS as human suffering. *Daedalus, 118*(2), 135–160.

Fattner, A. G., & Check, W. A. (1984). *The truth about AIDS: Evolution of an epidemic.* New York: Holt, Rinehart & Winston.

Fear of AIDS alters sex behaviour. (1987). *New Scientist, 1115,* 26.

Fee, E. (1988). Sin versus science: Venereal disease in twentieth century Baltimore. In E. Fee & D. Fox (Eds.), *AIDS: The burden of history* (pp. 121–146). Berkeley, CA: University of California Press.

Fee, E., & Krieger, N. (1993). Understanding AIDS: Historical interpretations and the limits of biomedical individualism. *American Journal of Public Health, 82,* 1477–1486.

Fisher, J. (1988). Possible effects of reference group-based social influences on AIDS—Risk behavior and AIDS prevention. *American Psychology, 43,* 914–920.

Fitzpatrick, J. D. (1988). AIDS is a moral issue. In L. Hall & T. Modl (Eds.), *AIDS: Opposing viewpoints* (pp. 32–36). St. Paul, MN: Greenhaven Press.

Fleming, W. (1964). Syphilis through the ages. In J. B. Youmens (Ed.), *Syphilis and other venereal diseases* (pp. 587–612). Philadelphia: Saunders.

Flora, J., & Carl, T. (1988). Reducing the risk of AIDS in adolescents. *American Psychology, 43,* 965–970.

Fox, D. (1986). AIDS and the American health policy: The history of prospects of a crisis of authority. *Millbank, 64*(Suppl. 1), 7–33.

Francis, D. P. (1988). Prospects for the future. *Death Studies, 12,* 598–607.

Frankenburg, R. (1989). One epidemic or three? Cultural, social and historical aspects of the AIDS pandemic. In P. Aggleton, G. Hart, & P. Davies (Eds.), *AIDS: Social representations, social practices* (pp. 21–38). New York: Falmer Press.

Frazier, J. (1922). *The golden bough: A study in magic and religion.* New York: Macmillan.

Friedland, G. (1989). Clinical care in the AIDS epidemic. *Daedalus, 118*(2), 59–83.

Friedman, S. R., Klienman, P. H., & Des Jarlais, D. C. (1992). History, biography, and HIV infection. *American Journal of Public Health, 82,* 125.

Fulton, R. (1990, March). *The future of AIDS.* Keynote address at the annual meeting of the Association for Death Education and Counseling, New Orleans, LA.

Fulton, R., & Owen, G. (1988). Death and society in twentieth century America. *Omega, 18,* 379–399.

Fumento, M. (1990). *The myth of heterosexual AIDS.* New York: Basic Books.

Gallo, R. C. (1989, October). My life stalking AIDS. *Discover,* pp. 31–36.

Garrett, L. (1994). *The coming plague: Newly emerging diseases in a world out of balance.* New York: Farrar, Straus & Giroux.

Garry, R. F., Witte, M. H., & Gottlieb, A. (1988). Documentation of an AIDS virus infection in the United States in 1968. *Journal of the American Medical Association, 260,* 2085–2087.

Gonda, M. (1989). The natural history of AIDS. *Natural History, 5,* 78–81.

Gostin, L. (1989). Public health strategies for confronting AIDS: Legislative and regulatory policy in the United States. *Gama, 261,* 1621–1630.

Gostin, L., & Curren, W. (1987). AIDS screening, confidentiality and the duty to warn America. *Journal of Public Health, 77,* 361–365.

Greeley, A. (1991). Religion and attitudes toward AIDS policy. *Sociology and Social Research, 75,* 126–132.

Grmek, M. (1990). *History of AIDS: Emergence and origins of a modern pandemic* (R. Maulitz & J. Duffin, Trans.). Princeton, NJ: Princeton University Press.

Gussow, Z. (1989). *Leprosy, racism and public health: Social policy in chronic disease control.* Boulder, CO: Westview Press.

Hall, L., & Modl, T. (1988). *AIDS: Opposing viewpoints.* St. Paul, MN: Greenhaven Press.

Harris, J., & Holm, S. (1993). If only AIDS were different. *Hastings Center Report, 23*(6), 6–12.

Hecker, J. F. (1846). *The epidemic of the middle ages* (B. F. Babingon, Trans.). London: George Woodfall & Son. (Original work published 1840)

Herek, G., & Glunt, E. (1988). An epidemic of stigma: Public reactions to AIDS. *American Psychology, 43,* 886–891.

Herzlich, C., & Pierret, J. (1987). *Illness and self in society* (E. Forster, Trans.). Baltimore: Johns Hopkins University Press.

Ho, D., Neumann, A. V., Perelson, A., Chen, W., Leonard, J., & Markowitz, S. (1995). Rapid turnover of plasma virions and CD4 lymphocytes in HIV-1 infection. *Nature, 373,* 123–125.

Hopkins, D. (1987). AIDS in minority populations in the United States. *Public Health Reports, 102,* 677–681.

Horton, M., & Aggleton, P. (1988). Perverts, inverts and experts: The cultural production of an AIDS research paradigm. In P. Aggleton, G. Hart, & P. Davies (Eds.), *AIDS: Social representations, social practices* (pp. 74–100). New York: Falmer Press.

Hourani, A. (1991). *A history of the Arab peoples.* Cambridge, MA: Belknap Press.

Imperato, P. J. (1989). Historical precedent and the obligation to treat AIDS patients. *Journal of Community Health, 14,* 191–195.

Institution of Medicine. (1986). *Confronting AIDS: Directions for public health, health care and research.* Washington, DC: National Academy Press.

Johnston, W., & Hopkins, R. (1990). *The catastrophe ahead: AIDS and the case for a new public policy.* New York: Praeger.

Jones, J. (1981). *Bad blood: The Tuskegee syphilis experiment.* New York: Free Press.

Judsen, F. (1989). What do we really know about AIDS control? *American Journal of Public Health, 79,* 878–882.

Kastenbaum, R. (1993). Reconstructing death in postmodern society. *Omega, 27,* 75–90.

Kastenbaum, R., & Aisenberg, R. (1976). *The psychology of death.* New York: Springer.

Kayal, P. (1985). "Morals," medicine, and the AIDS epidemic. *Journal of Religion and Health, 24*(3), 218–238.

Kelly, J., St. Lawrence, J., Smith S., Houd, H., & Cook, D. (1987). Stigmatization of AIDS patients by physicians. *American Journal of Public Health, 77*, 789–791.

Kennedy, R. E., & Fulton, R. (1995). *The emerging third state of the AIDS epidemic.* Unpublished manuscript.

Kerison, R. (1985, September 16). [Column.] *New York Post*, p. 4.

Kion, T. A., & Hoffman, G. (1991). Anti-HIV and anti-anti-MHC antibodies in alloimmune and autoimmune mice. *Science, 253*, 1138–1140.

Kleinberg, S. (1988). AIDS will transform the homosexual lifestyle. In L. Hall & T. Modl (Eds.), *AIDS: Opposing viewpoints* (pp. 206–211). St. Paul, MN: Greenhaven Press.

Klinghoffer, M. (1988). AIDS might be spread through casual contact. In L. Hall & T. Modl (Eds.), *AIDS: Opposing viewpoints* (pp. 47–52). St. Paul, MN: Greenhaven Press.

Kollar, N. (1982). *Songs of suffering.* Minneapolis, MN: Winston Press.

Kotarba, J., & Williams, M. (1990, August). *Adolescent intravenous drug users' informal health care network: The relevance of "friends." "Moms" for AIDS intervention.* Paper presented at the meeting of the American Sociological Association, Washington, DC.

Kovacs, J., Bueler, M., Dewer, R. J., Voges, S., Davey, R., Fallon, J., Polis, M. A., Walker, R. E., Salzman, N. P., Metcalf, J. A., Masur, H., & Lane, H. C. (1995). Increases of CD4 T lymphocytes with human immunodeficiency virus infection: A preliminary study. *New England Journal of Medicine, 332*(9), 567–575.

Kowalewski, M. (1990). Religious constructions of the AIDS crisis. *Sociological Analysis, 51*, 91–96.

Kushner, T. (1993). *Angels in America: A gay fantasia on national themes.* New York: Theatre Communications Group.

Lasagna, L. (1975). *The VD epidemic.* Philadelphia: Temple University Press.

Lee, R. (1987). *AIDS in America.* Troy, New York: Whitson.

Lester, C., & Saxxon, L. (1988). AIDS in the Black community: The plagues, the politics, the people. *Death Studies, 12,* 563–571.

Levine, A. (1992). *Viruses.* New York: Scientific American Library.

Levine, C., & Stein, G. (1994). *Orphans of the HIV epidemic: Unmet needs in six U.S. cities.* New York: The Orphan Project.

Lowell, A., Edwards, L., & Carroll, P. (1969). *Tuberculosis.* Cambridge, MA: Harvard University Press.

Lowey, G. (1988). Risk and obligation: Health professionals and the risk of AIDS. *Death Studies, 12,* 531–545.

Mahoney, S., & Cavenar, J. (1988). A new and timely delusion: The complaint of having AIDS. *American Journal of Psychiatry, 145,* 1130–1132.

Mann, J., Tarantola, D., & Netter, T. (Eds.). (1992). *AIDS in the world: A global report.* Cambridge, MA: Harvard University Press.

Marks, G., & Beatty, W. K. (1976). *Epidemics.* New York: Charles Scribner & Sons.

Martin, J. L. (1988). Psychological consequences of AIDS related bereavement among gay men. *The Journal of Consulting and Clinical Psychology, 56,* 856–862.

Martin, J. L., & Dean, L. (1993). Effects of AIDS-related illness on psychological distress among gay men: A 7 year longitudinal study. 1985–1991. *The Journal of Consulting and Clinical Psychology, 61,* 94–103.

Martin, J. P. (1988). Hospice and home care for persons with AIDS/ARC: Meeting the challenges and ensuring quality. *Death Studies, 12,* 463–488.

Mason, P., Olson, R., & Parish, K. (1988). AIDS, hemophilia and prevention efforts in a comprehensive care program. *American Psychology, 43,* 971–976.

Mays, V., & Cochron, S. (1988). Issues in the perception of AIDS risk and risk reduction by Black and Hispanic/Latina women. *American Psychology, 43,* 949–957.

McBride, D. (1991). *From TB to AIDS: Epidemics among urban Blacks since 1900.* Albany, NY: State University of New York Press.

McCombie, S. C. (1990). AIDS in cultural, historical and epidemiologic context. In D. Feldman (Ed.), *Culture and AIDS* (pp. 9–28). New York: Praeger.

McDonal, K., Jackson, J. B., Bowman, R. J., Polesky, H., Rhame, F., Balfour, F., Jr., & Osterholm, M. (1989) Performance characteristics of serological tests for human immunodeficiency virus test type 1 (HIV-1) antibody among Minnesota blood donors: Public health and clinical implications. *Annals of Internal Medicine, 1110,* 617–621.

McKusick, L. (1988). The impact of AIDS on practitioner and client: Mores for the therapeutic relationship. *American Psychology, 43,* 935–940.

McNeill, W. (1976). *Plagues and peoples.* Garden City, NY: Anchor Books.

Mooney, E. (1979). *In the shadow of the white plagues.* New York: Crowell.

Mulder, C. (1988). A case of mistaken identity. *Nature, 331,* 562–563.

Mullan, F. (1989). *Plagues and politics: The story of the United States.* New York: Basic Books.

Murphy, P., & Perry, K. (1988). Hidden grievers. *Death Studies, 12,* 451–462.

Murray, T. (1991). The poisoned gift. In D. Nelkin, D. Willis, & S. Parris (Eds.), *A disease of society: Cultural and institutional responses to AIDS* (pp. 216–240). NY: Cambridge University Press.

Musto, D. (1986). Quarantine and the problem of AIDS. *Millbank, 64*(Suppl. 1), 97–117.

Musto, D. (1988). Quarantine and the problem of AIDS. In E. Fee & D. Fox (Eds.), *AIDS: The burden of history* (pp. 67–85). Berkeley, CA: University of California Press.

Nelard, S. (1993). *How we die: Reflections on life's final chapter.* New York: Knopf.

Nelkin, D., & Gilman, S. (1988). Placing blame for devastating disease. *Social Research, 55*(3), 361–378.

Nelkin, D., Willis, D., & Parris, S. (Eds.). (1991). *A disease of society: Cultural and institutional responses to AIDS.* New York: Cambridge University Press.

Nicholson, W. (1919). *The historical sources of DeFoe's journal 4: The plague years.* Boston: Stafford.

Niven, R. (1987). The impact of AIDS on the chemical dependency field. *Advances in Alcohol and Substance Abuse, 7,* 3–14.

Nord, D. (1997). *Multiple AIDS-related loss: A handbook for understanding and surviving a perpetual fall.* Washington, DC: Taylor & Francis.

Oleske, J., Minnetor, A., Cooper, T. K., de la Cruz, A., Abdieh, H., Guerrero, I., Joshi, V., & Desposito, F. (1983). Immune deficiency syndrome in children. *Journal of the American Medical Association, 249,* 2345–2349.

Olson, J. (1989). *The history of cancer: An annotated bibliography.* New York: Greenwood Press.

Palca, J. (1986). AIDS in California: Proposition causes PANIC. *Nature, 323,* 384.

Panati, C. (1989). *Panati's extraordinary endings of practically everything and everybody.* New York: Harper & Row.

Panem, S. (1985, August). AIDS: Public policy and biomedical research. *Hastings Center Report,* 23–26.

Papathomopoulos, E. (1988). An attempt to commit suicide by contracting AIDS. *American Journal of Psychiatry, 145,* 765–766.

Patterson, J. T. (1987). *The dread disease: Cancer and modern American culture.* Cambridge, MA: Harvard University Press.

Paul, J. (1971). *A history of poliomyelitis.* New Haven, CT: Yale University Press.

Pearlin, L., Semple, S., & Turner, H. (1988). Stress of AIDS caregiving: A preliminary overview of the issues. *Death Studies, 12,* 501–517.

Perez-Stable, E. (1991). Cuba's response to the HIV epidemic. *American Journal of Public Health, 81,* 563–567.

Perrow, C., & Guillen, M. (1990). *The AIDS disaster: The future of organizations in New York and the nation.* New Haven, CT: Yale University Press.

Peterson, J. L., & Bakaman, R. (1989). AIDS and IV drug use among ethnic minorities. *Journal of Drug Issues, 19,* 27–37.

Peterson, J. L., & Marin, G. (1988). Issues in the prevention of AIDS among Black and Hispanic men. *American Psychology, 43,* 871–877.

Platt, J. (1987). The future of AIDS. *The Futurist, 21,* 11–17.

Poirier, R. (1988). AIDS and traditions of homophobia. *Social Research, 55,* 461–475.

Porter, D., & Porter, R. (1988). The enforcement of health. In E. Fee & D. Fox (Eds.), *AIDS: The burden of history* (pp. 97–120). Berkeley, CA: University of California Press.

Preston, R. (1979). *The dilemmas of care.* New York: Elsevier.

Preston, R. (1994). *The hot zone.* New York: Random House.

Quetel, C. (1990). *History of syphilis.* Baltimore: Johns Hopkins University Press.

Renovard, Y. (1978). The Black Death as a major event in world history. In W. Bowsky (Ed.), *The Black Death: A turning point in history?* (pp. 25–34). Huntington, NY: Krieger.

Richards, P. (1977). *The medieval leper and his northern heirs.* Cambridge, England: D. D. Brewer.

Richardson, D. (1988). *Women and AIDS.* New York: Routledge.

Rimer, S. (1995, August 30). Fear of AIDS grows among heterosexuals. *New York Times,* pp. A1, B2.

Robbins, R. S. (1981). Disease, political events and populations. In H. Rothschild (Ed.), *Biocultural aspects of disease* (pp. 153–176). New York: Academic Press.

Ron, A., & Rogers, D. (1989). AIDS in the United States: Patient care and politics. *Daedalus, 118*(2), 41–58.

Rose, J. W. (1988). An ethics of compassion: A language of division: Working out the AIDS metaphor. In I. Corless & M. Pittman-Lindeman (Eds.), *AIDS: Principles, practices and politics* (pp. 81–95). New York: Hemisphere.

Rosenberg, C. (1962). *The cholera years.* Chicago: University of Chicago Press.

Rosenberg, C. (1989). What is an epidemic? *Daedalus, 118*, 1–18.

Rosenbury, T. (1971). *Microbes and morals: The strange story of venereal disease.* New York: Viking Press.

Rothman, S. (1994). *Living in the shadow of death: Tuberculosis and the social experience of illness in American history.* New York: Basic Books.

Rothschild, H. (Ed.). (1981). *Biocultural aspects of disease.* New York: Academic Press.

Rundell, J., Paolucci, S., Beatty, D., & Boswell, R. N. (1988). Psychiatric illness at all stages of human immunodeficiency virus infection. *American Journal of Psychiatry, 145*, 652–653.

Sabatier, R. (1987). The global costs of AIDS. *The Futurist, 21*, 19–31.

Sapolosky, H., & Boswell, S. (1992). The history of transfusion AIDS: Practice and policy alternatives. In E. Fee & D. Fox (Eds.), *AIDS: The making of a chronic disease* (pp. 170–193). Berkeley: University of California Press.

Schneider, B. (1988). Gender, sexuality, and AIDS: Social responses and consequences. In R. Berk (Ed.), *The social impact of AIDS in the U.S.* (pp. 15–36). Cambridge, MA: Abt.

Schofferman, J. (1988). Cases of the AIDS patient. *Death Studies, 12*, 433–449.

Schwalbe, M., & Staples, C. (1992). Forced blood testing: Role taking, identity and discrimination. In J. Huber & B. Schneider (Eds.), *The social context of AIDS* (pp. 145–182). Newbury Park, CA: Sage.

Shannon, G., Pyle, G., & Bashsheer, R. (1991). *The geography of AIDS: Origins and causes of an epidemic.* New York: Guilford Press.

Shilts, R. (1987). *And the band played on: Politics, people and the AIDS epidemic.* New York: St. Martin's Press.

Shine, D., Moll, B., Emerson, E., Sprigland, H., et al. (1987). Serologic, immunologic, and clinical features of parenteral drug users from contrasting populations. *American Journal of Drug and Alcohol Abuse, 13,* 401–412.

Shufeldt, R. (1915). *America's greatest problem: The negro.*

Simpson, M. (1988). The malignant metaphor: A political thanatology of AIDS. In I. Corless & M. Pittman-Lindeman (Eds.), *AIDS: Principles, practices and politics* (pp. 193 208). New York: Hemisphere.

Slack, P. (1985). *The impact of plague in Tudor and Stuart England.* London: Routledge & Kegan Publishing.

Slack, P. (1988). Responses to plague in early modern Europe: The implications of public health. *Social Research, 55,* 433–453.

Smelser, N. (1963). *Theory of collective behavior.* New York: Free Press.

Smith, J. (1990). *Patenting the sun: Polio and the Salk vaccine.* New York: Free Press.

A social disease. (1985, September 14). *The Nation,* p. 196.

Sontag, S. (1978). *Illness as metaphor.* New York: McGraw-Hill.

Sontag, S. (1988). *AIDS and its metaphors.* New York: Farrar, Straus & Giroux.

Sorenson, J. L. (1991). Introduction: The AIDS drug correction. In J. Sorenson, L. Wermuth, D. Gibson, K. Choi, J. Guydish, & S. Batki (Eds.), *Preventing AIDS in drug users and their sexual partners* (pp. 3–17). New York: Guilford Press.

Stall, R., Coates, T., & Hoff, C. (1988). Behavioral risk reducation for HIV infection among gay and bisexual men: A review of results from the United States. *American Psychologist, 43,* 878–885.

Stoddard, T., & Reiman, W. (1991). AIDS and the rights of the individual: Toward more sophisticated understanding of discrimination. In D. Nelkin, D. Willis, and S. Parris (Eds.), *A disease of society: Cultural and institutional responses to AIDS* (pp. 241–242). New York: Cambridge University Press.

Sullivan, A. (1996, November 10). When plagues end. *New York Times Magazine*, pp. 52–62, 76–77, 84.

Tache, J., Selye, H., & Day, S. (Eds.). (1979). *Cancer stress and death*. New York: Plenum Medical Book Co.

Tarasoff v. Regents of the University of California. (1976). 131 *Cal Reporter*, 14, 551p. 2nd 334.

Thailand's double fear (AIDS alert might cause panic and loss of tourism). (1987). *New Scientist, 114,* 29.

Thompson, J. W. (1921). The aftermath of the Black Death and the aftermath of the Great War. *American Journal of Sociology, 26,* 565–572.

Titmus, R. (1971). *The gift relationship: From human blood to social policy.* New York: Random House.

Too much panic over AIDS? (1987). *Nature, 326,* 113–114.

Tuchman, B. (1978). *A distant mirror: The calamitous 14th century.* New York: Ballantine.

Twigg, G. (1984). *The Black Death: A biological reappraisal.* London: Barsford Academic and Educational.

Vachon, M. (1987). *Occupational stress in the care of the critically ill, the dying and the bereaved.* New York: Hemisphere.

Viney, L., Henry, R., Walker, B., & Crooks, L. (1992). The psychological impacts of multiple deaths from AIDS. *Omega, 24,* 151–163.

Waldork, D., Murphy, S., Lauderback, D., Reinarman, C., & Marotta, T. (1990). Needle sharing among male prostitutes: Preliminary findings of the Prospero project. *Journal of Drug Users, 20,* 309–334.

Walter, N. (1984). Learning to be a leper: A case study in the social constitution of illness. In E. Mishler, L. Amarsinghom, S. Hauser, R. Liam, S. Sherson, & N. Waxler (Eds.), *Social context of health, illness and patient care* (pp. 169–194). Cambridge, MA: Cambridge University Press.

Ward, J. W., Bush, T. J., & Perkins, H. A. (1990). The natural history of trans-fusion-associated infection with human immunodeficiency virus: Factors influencing the rate of progression to disease. *New England Journal of Medicine, 32,* 947–952.

Wass, H. (1986). Editorial. *Death Studies, 10,* iii–xiii.

Watkins, J. (1988). Responding to the HIV epidemic: A national strategy. *American Psychology, 43,* 849–851.

Weeks, J. (1989). AIDS: The intellectual agenda. In P. Aggleton, G. Hart, & P. Davies (Eds.), *AIDS: Social representations, social practices* (pp. 1–20). New York: Falmer Press.

Weisman, R. (1972). *On dying and denying: A psychiatric study of terminality.* New York: Behavioral Publications.

Williams, B. C. (1970). *Black Death and the maturing of man in the human side of history: Man's manners, morals and games.* Los Angeles: Manking Publishing Co.

Winiarski, M. (1991). *AIDS-related psychotherapy.* New York: Pergamon.

Winslow, C. E. A. (1943). *The conquest of epidemic disease: A chapter in the history of ideas.* Princeton, NJ: Princeton University Press.

Winslow, C. E. A. (1952). *Man and epidemics.* Princeton, NJ: Princeton University Press.

Wolf, L. (1972). *A dream of Dracula: In search of the living dead.* Boston: Little, Brown.

Yankauer, A. (1988). AIDS and public health. *American Journal of Public Health, 78,* 364–366.

Ziegler, P. (1969). *The Black Death.* New York: Harper & Row.

Zinsser, H. (1934). *Rats, lice and history: A study in biography.* Boston: Little, Brown.

INDEX